FOR

THE HEALTH

OF

A WOMAN

and

the Story

of

One Tree Hill

By Doctor David J L Brown M.D.

For the Health of a Woman

Dedications

This book is dedicated to my wonderful family past, present and future.
To my incredibly wonderful wife Cynthia and our fantastic children: Geraldine Sawyer (and husband Brent), Georgina (and fiancé Alex), Jenny (and page layout expert Byron) and James.

I dedicate this also to my parents and parents-in-law, who have all passed on, and all our sisters and brothers.

Of course, I am hopeful that this book will help all patients, both female and male.

Acknowledgments

This entire book project was made possible with kind and generous help from the following people.

The editor, David Wareham Evans, and his fantastic wife/assistant Lea Evans.
This couple donated time in the form of whole holidays, weekends and evenings, not only to discuss and edit but also to push and encourage me to take this project to completion.

My large and wonderful medical practice. All my patients, especially the women, who provided me with the incentive to write this book as a supplement to their annual medicals and to offer other methods in the prevention of injury-type disease.
A particular thank-you to Tammy Field for art supplies and to Mrs. Linda Carter for the inspiration to start "True Balance," and then this book.

Thank you Mr. Hugh Fuller for your guidance on legal matters.

I am not that bad at outdoor photography, but inside shots are my weakness. So, thanks to Kyle McLeod and his tremendous then-pregnant wife Genai, who both helped out with many sets and dedicated many days of their time. Their wonderful daughter Acacia will be proud.

Betty Jean Bonin was extremely generous in the donation of her riding manual, along with the illustrations that she provided. Horses, I know, must be extremely happy in your care. Many thanks also to Kathleen M. Massie, the expert rider in the photographs.

An extremely caring patient donated both her body and her time for Chapter 9 because of her sincere interest in the detection of early breast cancer. I know that everyone who reads this chapter will be grateful.

Finally, again I have to praise Cynthia, my wife, for her extreme patience, and for providing the love, care and catering that were so essential to the successful completion of this timely project. Sorry for your recurring dreams of cartoon characters!

Contents

Preface — A Young Boy's Adventure on One Tree Hill

Introduction
Falling Fears, Failing Sex, Fatigue, Fatness,

Fitness, and Facts on Menopause, as well as

The Warm Speculum: Special Care for a

Woman's Good Health

Chapter 1   Help! I'm Scared Stiff

Chapter 2   How To Look Younger Instantly

Chapter 3   Your Most Valuable Possession — You

Chapter 4   'Tunnel' Everything

Chapter 5   Human Landing Gear

Chapter 6   The Story of Osteoporosis — Part One —

How You Get Weak Bones

Chapter 7   The Story of Osteoporosis — Part Two —

The Way to Stronger Bones

Chapter 8   The Four — *and Three-thirds* — Seasons

Chapter 9   The Six-minute Self-breast Examination —

The Correct Way!

Chapter 10   Fish, Flavonoids and Feeding Facts on the

Body's Finest Fuels

Chapter 11   A Few More Ways To Kill Yourself

Chapter 12   How Can I Help You?

Chapter 13   More Important than Menopause —

Perimenopause

Chapter 14   Remedy Guide for Perimenopause — The

A to Z List

Chapter 15   Perimenopausal Sex — 'In a Nutshell'

Chapter 16   A Beginner's Guide to the *5x5 Mix* Injury

Prevention Activity System — Section

One — The Warm-ups

Chapter 17   The *5x5 Mix* — Section Two — The

Myotoners

Chapter 18   The *5x5 Mix* — Section Three — Stretch

and Pull

Chapter 19   The *5x5 Mix* — Section Four — Stability,

Balance and Posture

Chapter 20 The *5x5 Mix* — Section Five — Ground

Reflex and Landing Skills for Your Body

Chapter 21 The Big Ten Platinum Rules of Fall Injury

Prevention

Appendix — Five lists of many conditions that

increase the risk of falling

Glossary of Medical and Other Terms

Preface

Anyone who travels extensively through the countryside will, from time to time, hear about or see a hill with a single tree on it. To many people, an isolated tree on a hill stimulates the imagination, prompting them to ask why a hill or small mountain would have only one tree growing on it. How did that tree get on that hill? Was it planted by someone, and how did it survive, growing for dozens or even hundreds of years? If this lonely tree had been part of a forest, then obviously it was special to have survived so long. Growing on a hill for many years, resisting windstorms, heat waves, lightning bolts, vandalism, disease, and, of course, the many humans who, with some sort of profit in mind, just love to flatten the countryside, gives that tree a status that everyone should respect. For this reason, I have departed from the usual sort of prefatory remarks and decided to tell you a story — one that is not a fable but a true tale, and one that in a unique way provides the metaphor for the entire book. It is a story about a lone tree, a curious young boy, and a lesson learned for life.

A map of the route travelled by the young explorer described in the story below will help to illustrate the events that took place many years ago.

A Young Boy's Adventure on One Tree Hill

It all started years ago in a small, centuries-old village, deep in the Oxfordshire countryside in England. In full view of this tiny settlement was a nature lover's dream — rolling hills, mottled with every possible shade of green. Various types of forest dominated the landscape, but closer to the ground one could find many common, as well as rare, wild plants.

From the village, the landscape was familiar to everyone. Looking from 'left to right', the forest grew more dense, except in one place. Here there was a square-shaped open field, with seemingly nothing growing on it, except that is for a single tree. This hilly area was known by everyone in the village as 'One Tree Hill'. Anyone who cared about the village children would tell them not to go near that part of the hills. According to legend in that area, anyone who ventured near that sole tree would never be seen again! Moreover, village lore also told of a mysterious cottage nearby. No one knew who lived there, but it was reputedly the dwelling of an ogre!

One hot summer day, a curious boy of about 10 years of age decided that, despite the warnings, he was going to explore the forbidden area of the hills above the village. He set off early the next morning, on his bicycle, carrying his air gun and 'snake stick'. Being quite familiar with the dangers of the local wilderness, he would always carry a forked stick when hiking through any long grass or dense bush. This snake stick was used to push aside the long grass and bush twigs, then, if a snake appeared, he could use the forked end to pin its head safely to the ground, thereby avoiding a bite. Even at this tender age, the young boy had already realized that he did not want to shoot his air gun at anything living; he only used it for skill practice, using slate 'plates' as targets. Despite this belief though, he felt somehow secure with the air gun, which was similar to carrying a security blanket. He also felt somewhat like his western book hero, Davy Crockett, setting off into the wilds for yet another dangerous adventure. For true protection against any adversary, however, he would use his self-defense knowledge — learned from his weekly comic — and the snake stick as an extension of himself, keeping any opponent at a distance. Yes, this ten-year-old had to be tough growing up in a village where another boy was trying to fight him or a wild dog was likely to bite him. His favorite boys' comic showed a new martial arts self-defense move every week, which he keenly practised on his brother or on one of his tougher sisters.

Defense against a wild animal was an unusual feature, especially in a comic, but it was described for the benefit of its readers' safety (advanced thinking indeed on the part of the publisher!).

Anyway, armed with his knowledge of nature, his experience in watching out for dangers, and his skills in self-defense, the young boy had the confidence necessary to take on the lone tree on the hill, along with any legendary creatures that lived there as well.

It was only about a fifteen-minute bicycle ride to the base of the hills, but from there the trip had to be made on foot.

After hiding his bicycle in the dense bushes below the hills, the young boy made the long climb up through the bushes into a clearing. Despite his confidence and his snake stick, he nervously scanned the ground for adders, the only venomous snake known to the area. Once out of the bushed area, he was relieved because the ground visibility was better, but the unusual heat and glare of the early morning sun became the new hazard (sunglasses and sun block lotions were not carried by the average young naturalist and adventurer in the 1950s!).

At this side of the hills, the distinctive smell of juniper berries pervaded the air around, and scattered in the soft fine grass were patches of wild strawberries, small but thirst-quenching if one ate enough.

From this clearing, one could see the entire village below, as well as many square miles of open countryside. For the whole distance from this flora-rich region to his ultimate destination, the terrain would now change. To cross this clearing was similar to crossing a small minefield, for it was dotted with many sharp and sometimes ball-shaped lumps of glass-like flint, as well as many foot-sized holes that had been created by old rabbit burrows. Some of the larger flints were naturally hollowed out and lined with chalk, which created a skull-like appearance. To a stranger, this place would look like an extensive graveyard, because there were bleached rabbit skeletons mixed in with these small human-like 'skulls'.

It would take about forty-five minutes to cross this clearing, which would prove to be a tough hike on such a hot day, especially when there was no drinking water for miles around. Brave boy adventurers, of course, did not carry food or water on their expeditions!

His only thought at this point in the trek was to reach the 'caves'. These 'caves' were actually a large area of yew trees, which together formed a large canopy-like covering that extended across the peak of the hills, dropping down to a valley. These trees offered shade and a welcome coolness, and the ground was flat, spongy and smooth, a surface likely created by centuries of dead needlelike leaves dropping from the trees above. Darkness was the opposite extreme within this ancient forest, compared with the bright sunshine outside it. A powerful stillness existed here, so much so that any minute vibration or noise was easily detected. Even when walking, only rarely would a twig snap, but it created a momentary 'crack' that would echo loudly down through the 'caves'.

Despite the security of this silence, the young boy realized that he was not alone. It was not a noise that alerted him, but more of a feeling of a disturbance in the air. Each time that the feeling hit him — behind to the right, then to the rear from the left — he would rotate briskly to try to detect the cause for this new sensation. This feeling was explained by many of his village friends and relatives as one that announced the presence of a ghost. Despite this, he did not feel that this area was haunted, and was determined to locate the cause of this mystical sensation. With all his senses on alert, the 'battle' began. The air gun was lowered to the ground, but the snake stick remained at the ready. He knew that being super-relaxed was essential to success, so with slow, deep breaths he developed a calmness that matched that of the forest. With slow gentle rotations, he scanned in full circles; first the ground surface, then the tree trunks and the lower branches, and finally the patchy sky and the branches above. His eyes were adapted to the darkness by now, so seeing into the shadows was not difficult.

Time and time again that blur of a sensation was felt. But because of the calmness and patience that he had developed from observing nature over his few years of existence, he saw at the corner of his eye (at the edge of his visual field) a flare of white light flashing surprisingly close to his head. This occurred a few times, and over what seemed to be many minutes, but finally, following what seemed to be a pattern of movement, the apparition was seen on a floating away angle.

Instantly, the young boy knew exactly what was playing games with him: it was a barn owl! The bird was simply flying in and out in figure-of-eight paths that were tricky to follow, especially when the movement is silent.

Anyone who has seen a barn owl will remember how, more than any other bird, it has a remarkably ghostly look. Once recognized, the bird seemed to lose interest and disappeared in a flash.

Despite being a little weakened by this barn owl encounter, the drive to reach his destination spurred the ten-year-old to press on. The rest of the 'cave' walk was quiet, except for disturbing a few wood pigeons. Sounding like large books being slapped together down a hollow tunnel, pigeons flapping their wings in the total silence of this forest can still be a shock to even the most seasoned explorer.

Still carrying his stick and air gun, the edge of the yew forest was finally reached, heralded by the sparkling sunlight that pierced through the still dense branches. Suddenly, the full glare of the sun was temporarily blinding as he pushed through the last of the springy yew boughs into the open air. After a short rest, taking time to adapt to the sunlight, the continuation of the trek was seen to be downhill into a shallow valley. Underfoot was soft grass, and there were only a few scanty, low-lying bushes to get through; this was definitely the easiest portion of the adventure for energy consumption, and it seemed to offer the least risk of hazards.

Upon reaching the valley, and then going back uphill, a different type of forest, the much larger, beech woods, could be seen. This last type of densely treed slope led all the way to One Tree Hill. At this point, and despite the cool shade of the beech trees, the young explorer was hot and drenched with sweat because of the distance travelled and the heat of the day. The inner tremors, of course, added to the heat. One can imagine the thoughts running through this young boy's head. There he was, climbing up through this dark forest, and feeling brave as he clutched his air gun and snake stick. He was on the final approach to his destination!

Finally, he could see lights at the edge of the forest. He stopped to listen, and he wondered what fate awaited him, because this was where the legendary cottage stood — the cottage that was perhaps the dwelling of an ogre. From this cottage, a pathway led straight to that single tree, the mysterious one that was visible for miles around.

What was he going to do? Here he was, standing almost at the greatest legend of the village below. Was he going to finally find out the truth of One Tree Hill? He stood there frozen, unable to move a muscle — in the dark and alone! After a few more minutes, he was able to move hesitatingly ahead, but only for a few steps.

Suddenly, without any warning, out of the silence and darkness, there was an almighty crash! Not only did the noise paralyze him temporarily but also the appearance just ahead of him of a large dark shadow almost made his heart stop. For there, standing in front of him, was not an ogre but what appeared to be a large, giant beast of an animal. As his focus on the shadow improved, the young boy realized that this beast was not a beast at all, but a magnificent red deer stag! After all, this boy, as we know by now, was a student of nature, and he knew every plant, bird and animal around. This was a relief, but the boy remembers feeling quite humbled and insignificant before this large creature. They stared at each other for just a few seconds, then suddenly, as quickly as it had appeared, the stag took off, jumping over bushes and vanishing into the darkness. At this point, the boy backed up slowly, knowing that he had to get out of the beech woods. He turned, sprinted through the easily traversed beech-wood forest floor, broke through the bushes at the trees' edge, and then ran back down into the valley. The boy was still shaken because he had run so fast that it felt as if his feet were not even touching the ground. Feeling safer in the treeless valley, he now realized that it was an uphill climb back to the yew 'caves', and so the thirsty, tired youngster had to revert to a slow walk.

By now, the afternoon sun was already setting, so he decided, despite his initial confidence, to walk around the yew forest! The thought of going back through the now almost totally dark 'caves' was just too scary.

When the roundabout descent back into the dense bush was finally over, the young boy felt content and calm, stopping to relax for a short while to simply enjoy the quietness of the countryside. He would do this frequently on these expeditions, and often curious rabbits would hop up to him to see what he was doing. Just as his breathing settled to a slow rhythm, however, out of the bushes sprouted a sudden burst of what looked like tiny, darting shadows against the dark blue sky. What now? Startled, the young boy frantically jumped up, grabbing his air gun, because he knew that he had to move quickly. Although he was well aware what the 'shadows' were, nothing was going to stop his exit from this situation! There was no self-defense move for these 'foes', because they were bats! There were not that many of them, but the fear was that bats can get tangled up in your hair and into your clothing. This had been branded on his brain from his earliest years, so a bat encounter was always dreaded and to be avoided. With seemingly no time to think, down the hill the young boy fled, not even thinking about snakes (in his haste he left his snake stick behind) or other dangers. Bats! The thought alone was enough to make anyone run at top speed. Fortunately, he reached his bicycle with no more creatures jumping out at him. Just as he had left it, the bicycle was waiting to take him back down the final road — still a hill — to his home in the village. With his air gun in one hand, and the other on the handlebar of the bicycle, the young boy arrived safely after what had been an exciting and instructive adventure.

This young boy had always been timid and shy, despite his self-defense skills, and it was for this reason that he attempted this expedition by himself, because he was fearful of exposing his weakness to his friends. He never did tell anyone about this adventure; in fact, this is the first time this story has been told. If it did not occur to you during the telling of this story, I am sure that by now you will have realized that the young boy was *me!*

In looking back, I regarded the large red deer stag as a warning. As you already know, I never did have any intention of using my air gun, it was more of a security device. I remember the stag as a friend, who just simply appeared to say, "Keep away from this cottage ... and One Tree Hill," that is, avoid a risky situation if at all possible. A valuable principle was learned that day at One Tree Hill, one that I have never forgotten, and one that has served me well in both my personal life and in my professional career.

So, this is why I want you to think of this book as being like my real-life metaphor, the large red deer stag — a friend, and a warning to keep away from potential injuries. As described here, we can use knowledge, awareness and even wisdom, so that, at the end of every day, and despite many possible dangers, we can emerge injury free.

Remember, as well, that fear can be overcome, and, because fear can lead to injuries, body damage can be avoided with a 'warning' and with knowledge.

Throughout this book, many varieties of ways to avoid fractures and other physical damage (limbs, organs and head), along with an almost infinitesimal number of ways to hurt yourself, are described. The One Tree Hill story illustrates only a few principles, such as using surround vision, being aware of the possible directions of sinister occurrences (from below, above, etc), adapting your eyes to lighting conditions, balance combined with movement on hillsides, and so on.

I hope that you find this book informative, revealing and rewarding. Since the above adventure, many new experiences, based upon my numerous years of medical practice (along with specialized fitness activities), have allowed me to pass on to you the reader even more direct ways to help you to develop a healthy lifestyle and to avoid injuries. Please read on... and revise the ideas often.

A Young Boy's Adventure on One Tree Hill

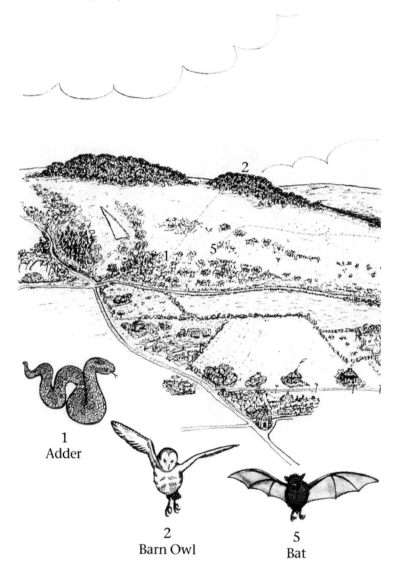

1
Adder

2
Barn Owl

5
Bat

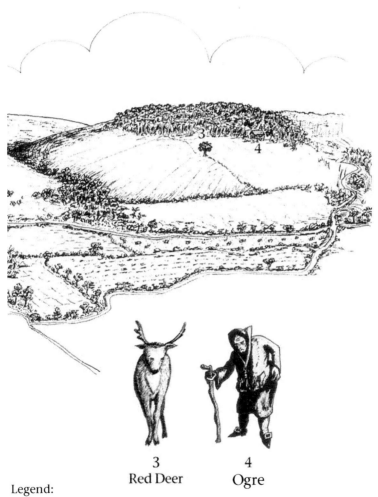

3
Red Deer

4
Ogre

Legend:

Path followed by the
boy on One Tree Hill

- - - - - - - - - -

Introduction

Falling Fears, Failing Sex, Fatigue, Fatness, Fitness,

and

Facts on Menopause

Good health and happiness are common wishes of all people, and both can be affected by the information offered here, along with aspects of women's diseases that are, at present, *missing health care directions.*

Are you really interested in preventing human disease, or in the latest treatment for such diseases? I am sure, because you are looking at a health-related book, that you would like to contribute to your health or to that of your loved ones in a positive way and by any method possible.

Every day, science is giving us new ways to prevent disease, including new drugs to combat such common diseases as the cancers that we all hear so much about and, of course, heart disease. One of the most common "diseases" to affect us all cannot be reduced in frequency or severity with a new pill *because there just is not one for it.*

In fact, this is one serious "disease" that medical science has little to offer us in the way of prevention — the misery of injuries!

Preserving good health, saving lives, and reducing suffering with a new prevention method is the purpose of the following chapters. The aim is not only to maintain body structure but also, in many cases, to improve body function and mental agility.

I would urge *every* woman over thirty years of age, all the way up to a ripe old age, to please understand these incredibly important facts:

- Breast cancer kills lots of women, but broken bones kill more!

- Most bone fractures are caused by falling!

- Falling is connected to many health changes that start before menopause!

In your hand, you are holding a single book for women, which can be thought of as three "books" in one, and it is expected that, just by following parts of the advice from each section, prevention of some common medical disorders can occur. Each consists of the following health sections:

Book one — A way to eat to prevent heart disease and cancer, along with advice on how to control many upsetting medical problems, are included here. These poor health conditions include obesity (unhealthy weight issues), severe tiredness (fatigue), depression, menopausal topics (along with sexual concerns), and much more. In addition, detailed self-breast examination is described.

Book two — An in-depth look at the "disease" of *fall injuries*, along with other injuries, is outlined. It shows ways of avoiding injuries in general, revealing special details on how *not* to break bones when you fall.

Ideas on preventing a fall are described, some of which are new, and some of which are not, but for *the first time ever, for use in everyday injury prevention*, you will be shown how to *land correctly* when falling over.

Book three — The basics of a home exercise system, called the *5x5 Mix*, are shown, using photographs and text to explain the reasons for the actions. This is a skill-training group of exercises on how to avoid the fall-type injuries; other benefits include improved fitness and weight loss.

Falling, tripping and slipping to the ground or tumbling downstairs are all common ways to hurt oneself. As already mentioned, falls often kill people.

In the study of disease, it has been found that more women die from fractures due to fragile bones than from the combination of all deaths from breast and ovarian cancers.

Because falls are common with elderly people, special training programs have been designed to attempt to reduce suffering or death from fall injuries. These programs are well planned and well delivered, but it is sometimes too late to help many people in this age group, because they are often frail, suffering memory loss, or have other medical problems. It is rare — seemingly unheard of — to find such fall prevention programs for younger people.

Anyone would agree that the best time to think about avoiding any disease (and injuries are classed as diseases) is to start the prevention program as soon as possible. *That is why this book exists!*

Think of the information in this book as a land safety program, akin to a water safety program. At swimming lessons, water safety is taught, and how to swim, of course, is the first lesson. This book uses the same concept, except it is for training in landing properly on the ground from a fall, thereby avoiding a possible injury or even death.

Swimming helps you to avoid drowning if you happen to fall in water. If you can swim, the chance of drowning is greatly reduced; therefore, if you can land *skillfully* from a fall, it goes without saying that the chance of fall injuries is greatly reduced.

Although this information is for the female sex, men should read it as well to help them to better understand the women in their lives. Even the section on breast examination should be practised by male partners, because some ladies cannot, for various reasons, do a self-breast checkup.

I consider this information to be a basic but missed vital step in the help needed to reduce injuries, especially of the falling type. Research is needed in this area of medicine; however, as with all new thinking, if you do not know the right people, it is extremely difficult to attract attention to a project. Another problem is, of course, the money. If money is not to be made from a project, there are not too many companies interested in financing a health system initiative.

The information shown here has been developed from my thirty years of medical experience in various medical specialties, including general practice, along with more than thirty years of knowledge in the methods of landing in a safe way from accidental or forced falls to the ground. Further experience was gained from teaching a regular class, called True Balance, which consisted of training mostly women in the *5x5 Mix* skills/fitness methods, along with detailed discussions on health issues.

In summary, this health book reflects much of my very existence, that is, my strong desire to prevent disease and to help my favorite species — women —   not only to survive illness but also to feel well!

The Warm Speculum: Special Care for a Woman's Good Health

I bet you are wondering what this is all about! If a job is worth doing, then it is worth doing right, and well. Helping to heal a health problem is still an art as well as a science. Careful and comfortable delivery of a doctor's health care can reach a diagnosis, as well as enable often safer treatment than simply just doing what is minimally necessary to reach the same end point.

I remember, many years ago, being taught how to examine the female pelvic organs. As he proceeded to examine a woman patient, I was horrified to see a gynecologist run freezing cold water over a metal speculum. Equally horrible for my newly qualified eyes was to see the patient squirm with the insertion of such an objectionably ice-cold device.

Working with a gynecologist who did not seem to care about the comfort of women was one alarming experience. Equally as bad as this actually gay male women's doctor were the many female midwives who would pour antiseptic solutions, straight out of the refrigerator, over the patient's pelvic outlet.

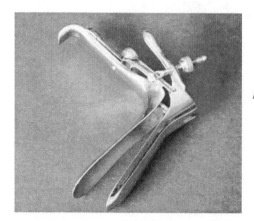

p-a A steel vaginal speculum

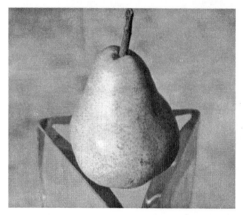

p-b This pear resembles the shape of the human uterus

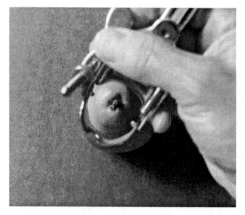

p-c This shows how a vaginal speculum is used to open the vagina to reveal the neck of the womb (the cervix). The pear represents the womb. The stalk shows where the fine brush is inserted into the cervix when taking a Pap test.

Can you imagine being in active labor, your legs are wide apart, you are naked from the waist down, and then someone pours ice-cold liquid over your private parts.

I am now 'famous' in my practice for warming all cold objects that have to be inserted into a human body. On one occasion, I was temporary entertainment for a fairly large crowd of customers in a hair salon. It was an uncommon event for me to accompany my wife to this popular Saturday morning women's beauty retreat.

One of the receptionists, a patient at the time, looked up and acknowledged my presence by saying in a loud voice,
"Hi, Doctor Brown, I'm glad you could make it too."
With that comment, one of the hair stylists perked up and said,
"Hey, is that the doctor who warms the speculum for your Pap test?"
(It is well-known how much information is passed around hair salons, especially private stuff!)
With a blush, I proudly agreed that it was I who was the warmer of all speculums, for all women.

Why was I proud? Not just because I was made to feel comfortable among mostly strangers concerning such a delicate topic but also because a little thing such as the warming of a speculum meant so much to a patient, even

though it was not medically necessary to get a good
scientific result.

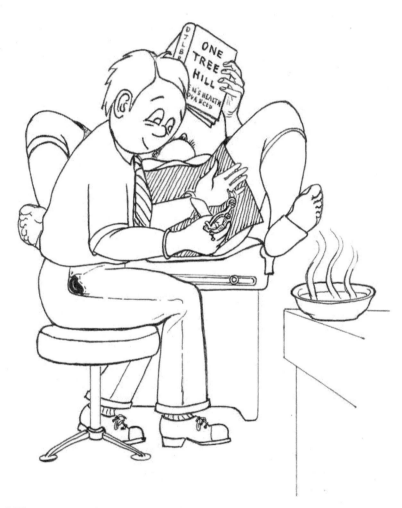

*p-d The warm speculum in action. The patient is quite comfortable reading her
book on the One Tree Hill story (Preface) because she knows the speculum will
be warm.*

For the sake of completeness, I must illustrate the use of the word "safer" when commenting on treatment being done in a proper way.

In an unfortunate incident, many years ago, a more experienced female gynecologist than me intervened when I was doing a D & C (an operation in which the lining of the uterus is scraped). Telling me I was being too gentle, she pushed me one side and took over. This doctor was extremely heavy-handed in everyday life, which put her at a disadvantage when doing a D & C. With her unnecessarily aggressive technique, she promptly pushed the operating tool right through the uterus, causing a hemorrhage. An emergency hysterectomy was necessary to save this woman's life.

Here are three messages for new health care providers:

First message — Do whatever it takes to help heal the sick, to prevent injuries, and to make them feel well.

Second message — Treat gently and safely, and show respect for all people, regardless of whether they are rich, poor, famous, or seemingly just a nuisance.

Third message — Remember that current thinking or methods of treatment will tomorrow, or in the near future, be "old school." When helping the sick and others in need of health advice, try to help by thinking of any safe way, whether it be ancient, modern, or possible treatment tested as safe but not necessarily accepted by those we think of as experts in the medical world. Historically, we know that professional guidelines change, often annually, so obviously they are not the final word in treatment advice. In other words, try not to be the most up-to-date scientific doctor when trying to help people's minds, bodies and families. The art of medicine is still needed and all of us have a lot to learn.

Please read this book critically, and please help people to understand what I am trying to help them with in the rest of this book. We, as health administrators, are not always the best at getting the health points to stick (time being one of our main brakes).

I hope, at least, to show everyone that an injury is a serious cause for ill health, and even death, and that it is a common disease that needs more medical attention, so that we doctors can regularly give preventive advice, just as we do for other diseases such as breast cancer.

The four illustrations (p-a, p-b, p-c and p-d) shown above will help to reduce the need for you to have to imagine what the Pap test is and how it is performed. A definition of the Pap test will be found in the Glossary at the end of this book.

Chapter 1

Help! I'm Scared Stiff

This information is as important as a breast examination!

Falling

"Your blood pressure is higher than usual today," I pointed out, in a somewhat surprised tone, to my patient Mrs Flynn, during what was *supposed to be* a routine medical visit. This woman was not really ill that day, but this did turn out to be an extremely important appointment.

"Do you feel OK? You certainly look OK", I asked, noting her looking anxiously at the view outside the window of my second-floor examining room.

"Honestly, I am taking my tablets," she said, "but it's the ice, you see, and my friend just broke her arm when she slipped over just yesterday. I'm scared silly that I'm going to fall over and break a bone. Sometimes, I hate these winters over here," she remarked, in her still strong Liverpudlian accent (originally she had lived in Liverpool, England).

"You really are scared, and that is making your blood pressure go up. You are afraid of falling, but I bet your blood pressure would come right down to your usual levels if I could take away that fear," I told her confidently (see cartoon 1-a).

This patient, who was in her late sixties, had a problem common at this age, in that she was afraid of breaking bones. We spent some time talking about falling over, and I explained to her that it was possible to experience a fall but not break a bone or even get hurt. The important thing was that she became more relaxed just simply talking about her worries and listening to details of what preventive measures are possible, and her blood pressure actually settled to normal.

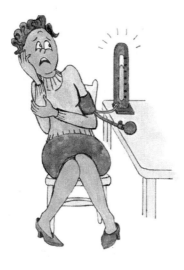

1-a This woman is so afraid of being hurt by a fall to the ground that her blood pressure is higher than usual

Why was this appointment so important? Because it was then that I decided to share with you all the *secrets* of the ways that you can avoid an injury when falling. These *secrets* are not really secrets, but they are systems of injury prevention that are not known to the average person. The combination of the chapters in this book make up these so-called *secrets*.

The above patient, although healthy, is one of the many who are afraid of falling. Although not old, she was extremely wise, in that, although she felt well, she realized that falling can cause serious health problems. The average person who feels healthy does not think that they are prone to falling injuries. Yet, in the single week prior to my writing this chapter, there were four separate incidents in which four healthy ladies all fell down the stairs! Fortunately, there were no deaths, but they were all left with some sort of an injury, including broken bones. It was interesting that the fittest of the four ladies, a yoga expert, was the least injured, although since then she has fallen down the stairs again and broken her wrist. It is a fact that people who fall over tend to have repeat falls, and, as illustrated here, yoga, just like many other fitness systems, does not include the teaching of skills designed to spread the forces of a fall to the ground. It was fortunate that these patients were relatively young, aged between 30 and 50 years of age. One can only imagine what would have happened if they had been much older.

It is not just doctors who notice that these injuries are a serious health concern. Various government health statistics, and groups of people interested in health issues, have also shown that injuries kill more women each year than breast and ovarian cancer combined! I repeat this fact purposely because it is so important.

Injury problems are worsening as health issues!

If we look once again at the types of injuries that are causing these deaths, government records reveal that fractures from *falling over are the most common culprits.*

Many health centers, including exercise gymnasiums, now have extremely good programs that teach the prevention of falling, as well there is lots of research on this topic that has been carried out by specialized health practitioners, including engineers who design and perform this research. Their goal, of course, is to attempt to reduce injuries and therefore save lives. Many of these programs developed for injury prevention are designed with only elderly people in mind. As you will see, when you peruse the rest of the chapters of this book, we are dealing not only with the prevention of falling but also with that *next extremely important stage after falling — the landing!*

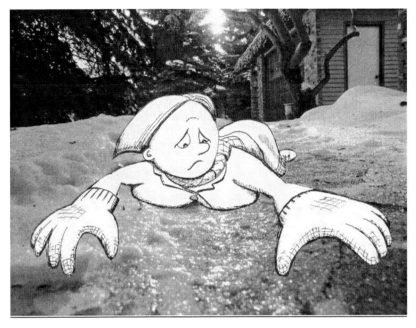

1-b A fall on ice can be humiliating as well as painful

Landing and Impacting

So, despite our efforts with fall *prevention* programs, including the addition of tai chi to the various exercise routines that are included in these clinics, *people still do fall and collide with a surface of some sort.* It would be ideal if people at a higher than average risk of falling over (see the Appendix section at the end of this book) could be taught to land in such a way that injury could still be prevented.

In summary, fall prevention programs are becoming more available, and they are certainly providing an excellent way to assess *older* people and help them to reduce their risk of dying from injuries; however, *preventing* falls is not always possible, and so understanding the information shown in many of the following chapters is necessary, *preferably* when you are young, to help you to understand the act of *correct landing* from a fall, thus avoiding an unpleasant collision with a surface or an object.

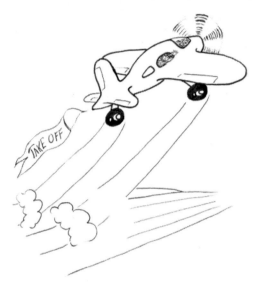

1-c This information takes off in the world of injuries where other books finish. The landing from a takeoff is also dealt with.

This book takes off where some sources of information end in providing advice on personal injury prevention. Illustration 1-c emphasizes this point. It is extremely important to understand everything about the life-threatening disease of falling-type injuries, and to know about skills that, when mastered, prevent, or certainly reduce, the severity of injuries sustained in a fall.

Developing your injury prevention skills as early as you can will give you rewards more important than any material possession that you could ever own. You will never be too old (depending on your health, but at least up to 80 years of age) to learn the skills and ways to avoid fall fractures, but the sooner you learn these methods the more you will minimize your lifetime risk of becoming a victim of this major disease.

If you, the reader, have any interest in the prevention of disease, and I am sure that you do, complete your knowledge by starting right now. Realize that injuries do maim and kill, and therefore have to be stopped.

Today, start the process of understanding surround vision, human landing gear, and the *5x5 Mix* exercises, so that the process of preservation, with the undoubted improvement of your health, can begin *now!*

Chapter 2

How To Look Younger Instantly

To look younger is highly desired by most women and men, and the older we get the more we want to look as well as feel younger. One of the reasons for this is that age, for many of us, brings so many undesirable changes in our bodies: symptoms such as aches and pains, reduced energy, reduced strength, and of course the development of various diseases. Along with this, our appearance usually deteriorates in a variety of ways. Because of the limitations of this book (it is, after all, about injuries), aging cannot be dealt with as a complete topic, but bone health, stature, balance and movement are certainly relevant to the topic of injury prevention, and so these will be included in some detail.

Whether standing, walking or sitting, a good upright posture makes you look much younger, and it is healthier for your skeleton and for your internal organs.

Here is a simple test. First, make sure that your hair is away from your neck, then look in a mirror in a slouched position, that is, standing, head and shoulders dropping forward. Judge your appearance! Now, simply *stand tall*, that is, spine straight, tummy and chin tucked in, shoulders pulled back as if you were standing to attention, and take in a deep breath. Note the amazing difference!

The above test is easy to perform, unless you have an abnormal spine. The difficult task is to get yourself to stand tall regularly, eventually achieving and maintaining an ideal upright posture. Below, there are ideas on how to improve your posture.

"Doctor, how can I improve my posture?" This question is not a common one for patients to ask their health practitioners, but I have been surprised that this question has been asked by relatively young patients. But more patients should be concerned about their upright posture, because it is important for general well-being, including bone health and injury prevention. As every year passes and you get older, caring for your upright posture (spine) becomes more important.

The assessment of the issues of balance and posture should begin in your health practitioner's office: first by a discussion of this aspect of health, followed by an examination of the skeleton.

Although they cannot be separated, posture with spinal care, balance and movement will be considered separately for ease of discussion.

The head is a heavy structure, and so, if it is aligned incorrectly for the postures necessary in many sports and other activities, your balance will be thrown off!

Please note again that your head position, if not held high, can make you look older!

Let us look at posture in more detail. The definition of posture, according to *Webster's Third New International Dictionary*, is the "relative arrangement of the different parts esp. of the body: the characteristic position or bearing of the body or that assumed for a special purpose...."

The term posture is used in many moving arts and sports. Yoga, along with some martial arts, has copied some *forms* that are seen in nature, and called them *postures*. Some examples of these are the Crane styles, Cat stances, Locust positions/postures, and the Lotus position. The various positions in martial arts are called defensive postures, because they are known to be balanced and useful in a fighting situation.

Good postures in all sports are essential, because they allow more perfect movement (this feels better for the participant, looks better, and is less tiring). In many movements, in sports as varied as dancing, gymnastics and horse riding, poor posture can be dangerous. In horse riding, for example, to be good at all riding techniques, including trotting and jumping, remaining in an upright posture on the horse is extremely important, for both safety and effect. This good riding posture is essential for the balance of both the rider and the horse (see photographs 2-a and 2-b).

2-a After her initial safety check, this rider is observing her horse's readiness to be mounted. She is showing the ideal grip of the rein and saddle horn prior to mounting the horse.

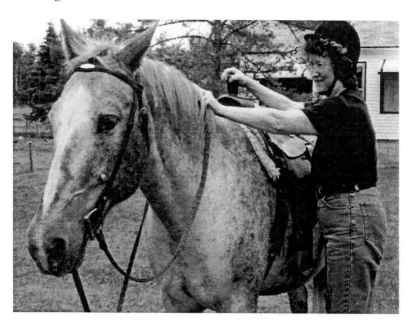

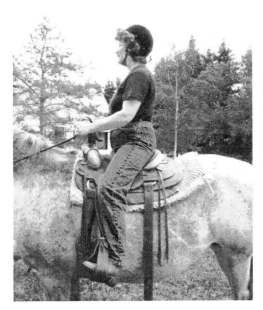

2-b A riding expert is demonstrating her posture on her stationary horse. When riding, protective gear such as a riding helmet is essential, other gear should be secure as well though, and skills in landing from a fall are highly recommended. (Photographs 2-a and 2-b courtesy Betty Jean Bonin from her riding manual, "Introducing the Horse".)

Now, back to good posture, as related to your health. Knowledge of good posture, as you will see, is important for health because it improves balance, which in turn helps to avoid fall injuries and is necessary to prevent the worsening of spinal deformities. Once you understand the disease of osteoporosis, you know that bone softens as it loses strength. When this happens in the vertebrae (spine), there is a tendency for the spine to tilt forward, causing a deformity called a kyphosis, which slowly gets worse unless treatment is started early in the disease. This spinal curvature causes a number of health problems. The affected person becomes noticeably shorter, they might feel back pain, they lose spinal strength, and the internal organs become compressed, so that the lungs, the heart, the intestines and the kidneys cannot function to their best capacity. The ability to rest, to move and to react with quick reflexes is also affected. A person with this disorder, depending on the severity, will tell you many more bad things about this preventable disease.

Diagram 2-c, figure 3, shows what is meant by a good upright posture. Putting it into words, it means that your spinal column should be in the natural upright position and your head should be over the vertical spine (aligned with the pull of gravity). Assuming that the abdominal muscles are working correctly, you should have your abdomen pulled in, so that, when seen from a side view, and with the spine straight, the ear is aligned with the hip joint.

Another way of describing it is that the center of the head is aligned with the heart and the hip joint (again looking from the side). The above description refers to the upright posture, although good postures, as already mentioned, can be achieved in this way while kneeling or sitting, or in the various postures of the sports mentioned above. Maintaining a flexible spine is the other goal of most exercise systems and sports. The ability to fully flex to the front or side, and then return to a straight upright posture, is practised regularly.

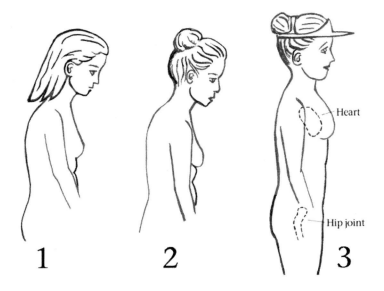

2-c (1, 2 and 3) In figure 1, the girl's long hair hides the forward curve of the neck. Figure 2 shows her hair held away from the neck, revealing and exaggerating the head forward position. In both diagrams, please note her drooping breasts and creased abdominal surface. As shown in figure 3, however, wearing a peaked cap is one way to encourage an improved posture. With a more upright position, the abdominal cavity can reach optimum volume, enabling the contents to spread inward. This permits the visible surface skin and fat to flatten out. Please notice, in this excellent standing posture from the side view, how the ear is aligned with the heart and the hip.

An important factor to be aware of is that in any of the perfect posture positions, for example, the upright posture, most muscles should be relaxed. If you have good tone in the abdomen, the muscles here will hold the intestines against the spine — much like a sac of water — giving it excellent support. In this position, the muscle tone in the legs should be minimal when standing still.

So, when you are analysing your perfect upright posture in the mirror, purposely relax your shoulder and jaw muscles, as well as any of the other muscles that are unnecessary for active movement. Along with nice deep breaths, this good habit can make all the difference in how you feel: *calm, comfortable and relaxed.*

Your Balance Point

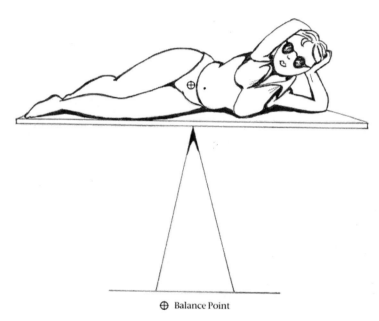

⊕ Balance Point

2-d This woman is exposing too much skin to the sun's rays, but only for a short time. She is relaxing on a board that is on a pivot, just to demonstrate the body's balance point. When her balance point is exactly over the peak of the support, the board will not tilt.

Gravity pulls us all, including all objects, toward the center of the earth. Everything that is solid has a center of gravity, including us human beings. When we are in the standing position, our center of gravity is a point low in the abdomen, level with a point about 4 cm below the navel (tummy button). If we were to lie across a balancing scale, so that we were not tilting one way or the other, the pivot of the scale would be at the center of gravity, we can call this the balance point of the body (see diagram 2-d).

The balance point is in a constant position when standing still in the upright position; however, when moving or lying down, *this point changes position.* To illustrate this, the following diagrams show the various changing positions. This central point of the body varies even more when two moving people or bodies are connected in some way. Two examples of this are a horse and rider and pairs in skating.

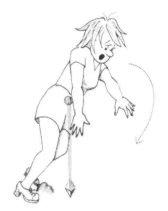

2-e Unsteady Freddi is falling forward because her balance point is not over either foot or any other support. Her left foot would have been placed under her balance point in a reflex way, but a rock on the ground prevented this natural walking reflex action.

Why is this balance point important in injury prevention? Well, this point of the body is important because, if it moves out of alignment with the feet, a fall can result. Illustration 2-e demonstrates this, in that, as the balance point moves ahead of the feet, gravity pulls the upper body down toward the ground, resulting in a fall. The balance point should not be confused with the balance center in the brain. The inner ear, the cerebellum part of the brain, works with other parts of the nervous system to let you know where your body is positioned in relationship to your environment. These brain centers are exercised in many parts of the exercise system, as are the inner ear organs of balance.

The technical term for the inner ears is the labyrinths. These are tiny tubes, set in the bone of the skull, that act just like small spirit levels. Within each ear, there are three of these tubes, curled into a circular shape. Each circular tube, officially called a semicircular canal, is arranged in a different direction to the other, so that three directions of movement can be monitored and reacted to by the brain, that is, the person. The movements referred to are the rotations or tilting of the body. These rotations can be described simply as (see diagram 2-f): 1) spinning (the red arrow); 2) side tilts (the yellow arrow); and 3) forward with back tilts, or rolling forward/backward (the blue arrow)

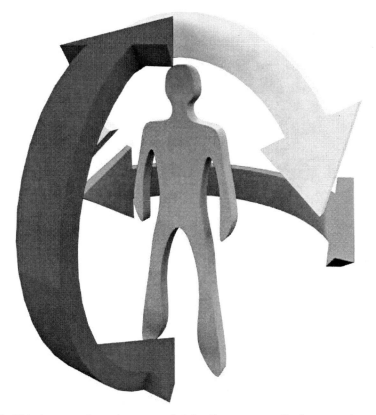

2-f This human shape is surrounded by three arrows. Each arrow demon-strates the directions of body movement (rotation) detected by the inner ear. Assuming that the person is facing forward, the front blue arrow (up/down) shows back or forward tilt motion, the red arrow wrapping around the back (as if a belt were closing in from behind) refers to vertical rotation of the body, and the yellow arrow over the top of the head refers to the lateral tilting or side-to-side movements. These arrows also indicate the three basic ways that the body can fall to the ground from a standing position.

There are, of course, tilts and rotations in between these three basic body movements, such as tilting forward to the right or left. In fact, if you imagine yourself inside a sphere, such as a giant ball, and imagine that ball being rolled around in random directions, you can see that there are an infinite number of directions in which your body could be rotated or tilted. The human body can recognize these multiple angles of rotation by combining the detecting abilities of the three semicircular tubes or canals, both left and right.

To exercise each of these left and right labyrinths, your activity system has to include rotation in the three directions (see the rolling log, tin cans and spinal rocks types of exercise in the *5x5 Mix* chapters).

Being aware of the balance point, along with having good posture control, helps you to move your balance point to a safe new position when you change body positions. By using this reflex when you do suddenly change position, you will automatically place a limb under the balance point, thereby preventing a fall. The average person does alter balance naturally to adjust to a body position change, but by using the methods outlined in the exercise system and by practising correcting your posture the reflexes are sharpened.

Walking

Both walking and standing can be described in so much detail that this entire book could have been written about human locomotion. This section on movement, therefore, has to be covered briefly in just a few sentences.

From the upright position, walking is simply moving your balance point forward, placing your one foot under this point to take the weight of your body, and then transferring the balance point forward again, placing your other foot under the new balance point center. This action creates a forward movement. The same activity in reverse will create a backward walk. If the balance point is moved forward (or backward), but the foot is not able to catch your body weight, a fall will result (see illustration 2-e).

As mentioned above, normal walking involves many complex nerve, muscle, joint and brain actions that are too complex to mention here.

There are many diseases that cause abnormal movements and affect walking abilities. As with simple walking, there is too much information about this topic to discuss it here. Imagine describing running, along with other complex movements. They are mentioned only to suggest further reading. If you need more detail or information on normal walking, as well as on the diseases of movement, you are advised to consult books on physiology, neurology and orthopedics.

10 Ways To Improve Your Posture

1)   Using a straight post, a wall or a straight pole (a broomstick) to rest against your back, so that it simultaneously touches your lower back (near the tailbone), your upper back, and the back of your head, adjust the rest of your body, so that it feels relaxed (see photographs in the *5x5 Mix* exercise chapters).

2)   Check your image daily in a reflective surface, such as a mirror or store window, to ensure that you are maintaining your body position.

3)   Practise the posture with balance exercises at least twice a week.

4) Practise abdominal and neck strengthening exercises every fourth day.

5) As a challenge and a reminder, try balancing a small bag of flour or a book on your head while walking or simply squatting down (see exercise chapters). Carry a backpack, weighing about 20 pounds, when walking. The straps should pull your shoulders back helping to correct your posture.

6) Wearing a back or abdominal brace will encourage you to both stand and sit straight up. If you do not keep in a continually upright posture, the edge of the back brace will dig into your groin or lower ribs!

7) Join an activity that stresses/encourages a good upright posture, such as yoga, ballroom dancing, tai chi, horse riding or ice skating. You could even join the armed forces!

8) Ask your spouse or a friend to comment on your posture regularly. Encouraging comments, such as "head up," "back straight," "chin in" or "stand tall," should be uttered by these observers when they notice you slouching. If you regularly wear a cap with a long peak, or a hood that hangs over the forehead, you will have to stand in an upright stance to be able to see straight ahead — a good trick to make good posture a good habit (see illustration 2-c).

9) Avoid using a pillow when sleeping, unless you are lying on your side. (Check with your doctor if you have a medical condition that requires a pillow, an example would be a hiatus hernia. For this condition, however, it is the whole upper body that has to be raised up, not just the neck.)

10) Hang upside down, using an inversion table. This reversal of gravity treats your body as if it is a pendulum,

which will in effect pull your body straight. (Check with
your doctor or with a fitness expert, as well as looking at
the instructions for the inversion device, before attempting
upside-down exercises.)

Chapter 3

Your Most Valuable Possession — You!

There is a price on your head; in fact, there is a price on your whole body! Just how much are our health and our bodies worth in money?

Jenni, Freddi's sister (illustration 3-a), is curious as to why she has been used as a model for this book, and she is also wondering what she is worth. How do we put a price on a human being? Try to guess what you are worth in money.

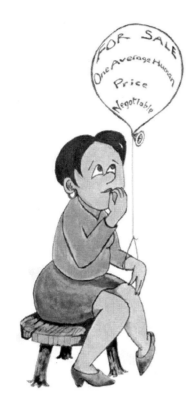

3-a Jenni is curious about what the balloon means — 'For Sale — One Average Human Price Negotiable' — What do you think you are worth in money?

Health practitioners and government departments often emphasize the cost of illness. For example, these economic health experts, who study health from the financial aspect, might express certain diseases as costing *x* units of currency (dollars, eurodollars or pounds) to treat yearly. Even the cost of being overweight is calculated as a cost to each country's health budget, and both heart disease and cancer are frequently expressed in monetary terms.

Grouping all injuries together, and classifying them as diseases, enables experts to track injuries, which then allows comparisons to be made among all diseases. We cannot assume that cost and seriousness are the same thing, but they are a guide to understanding the impact of illness on a nation.

When we do compare the costs of illnesses, however, it is surprising that injuries can *cost more than cancer* to assess and treat in most developed countries. The cost of looking after people medically for their injuries is interesting as well as important, but because injuries are increasing in number, and because the survival rate from cancers and heart attacks is improving with modern treatments, it is of the utmost importance that we implement as many ways as we can to prevent suffering and death from trauma of any kind.

There are many reasons why everyday products, as well as diseases, get attention of any kind: one of the biggest reasons for this is *advertising*. Clever advertising can sell almost anything to almost anyone. Most people are aware that products of almost any kind are bought every day; however, money is often spent on useless items, just because of excellent advertising.

Every day, health facts and treatments are advertised in many ways, by publication in magazines and newspapers, by way of television and radio commercials, and by postings on the Internet. Word-of-mouth promotion has a powerful effect on many people as to the meaning of diseases and how to treat them. Whether right or wrong, health remedies are passed on from family to family, or from often unqualified salespeople to an unsuspecting public. Some readers might have noticed expertly prepared documents on health issues displayed in hospitals and other medical facilities.

Conditions such as heart disease and cancer are common, and justifiably they both get *media attention* and *financial attention*; moreover, the combination of these two mighty forces is certainly associated with improved treatment success.

But the big question is this: Why are injuries not as well advertised as such well-known disorders as breast and other cancers, diabetes and heart attacks?
One answer to the above question boils down to money, the lack of which is the root of so many world problems.

Another factor that explains the 'quietness' of injuries is that they are not a single problem, and are not therefore easily identified as a disease, even by many doctors.

On behalf of all world injury prevention experts, it is hereby declared that trauma to the body is a top cause for human misery that must be controlled as much as any other disease!

Successful organizations are extremely good at selling their products because they hire top-quality firms to create catchy commercials; however, although governments also pay for the production of injury advertising that is informative, their products *lack the ability to attract curiosity.* When twenty-five people were asked at medical interviews in my own medical office if they could remember a television commercial about diarrhoea, they not only remembered finding the advertisement funny but could also recite the script almost word for word. Those same people were then asked if they could remember a frequently shown injury awareness television commercial. Out of the twenty-five questioned, *not one* could recollect ever seeing or hearing such an advertisement!

It is this doctor's wish that a relatively neglected, serious medical problem could be 'sold' to people, for the sake of awareness and prevention, in just the same way that commercial products are promoted, with *money, art and style!*

Keeping with the topic of selling for profit, fitness systems and weight control cannot be left out, for it is amazing what can be sold to the public in this segment of health. Whether a dietary aid or an exercise method is good or not, it will sell for at least a while if it is well advertised. A catchy name and a new way to get to people with a scientific-sounding explanation work to sell almost anything. If a health product prolongs life or improves the quality of life, it obviously would be worth the money spent to acquire it. Injury prevention methods deserve both expense and much effort being spent on them, and should certainly receive as much or more than most other existing health products, including drugs, exercise equipment and methods to reduce excess body fat.

Before looking at the types of problems that fall injuries can cause for those who suffer them, we should look at how experts group or classify these 'diseases'.

You can see that the "injury tree" (see diagram 3-c) shows a large variety of injury types, each branch representing the many different ways that you can get hurt or killed. It also represents the many diseases that you are supposed to avoid to prevent pain, suffering and death, and, of course to help *you, along with your government, to save money!*

We will now zero in on the branches of our injury tree, which looks at falls onto the ground and other hazardous surfaces.

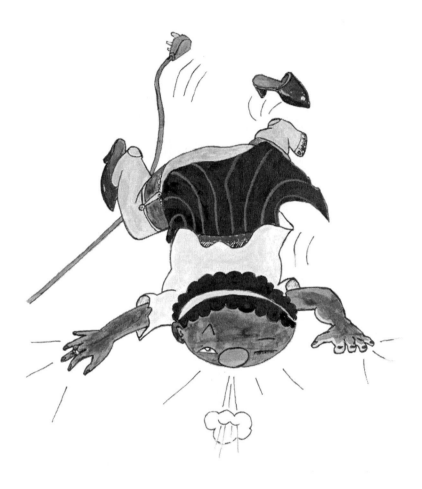

3-b Tripping over a cord is a common type of fall inside the home

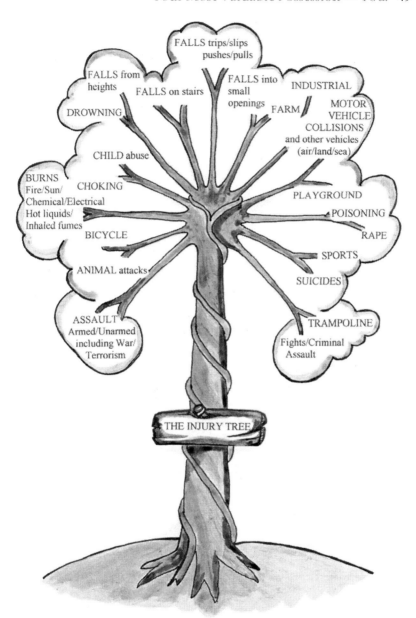

3-c The Injury Tree shows the many classes of injuries that can maim or kill a human. Wrapping itself around the trunk of the tree is a thick ivy stem, tempting a person to climb to the top of the tree. It is possible to avoid many of the injury types shown in the tree branches. Do not put yourself at the risk of unnecessary suffering!

Falling over can belong to the deliberate group of injuries, to the unplanned group of injuries, or to a mixture of both. The unplanned but forced fall describes the mixed group of falls, an example being when you are *accidentally* pushed over, that is, there is no intention of forcing you to fall.

As you can see from the "injury tree", there are four main types of fall:
- Falls from the standing position (either when still or in motion), the *slip, trip, pushover/pullover group*
- Falls on *stairways*
- Falls from *various heights*
- Falls through *narrow openings*

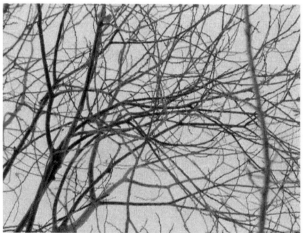

3-d *These willow tree branches divide in every direction possible; they twist, bend and push against each other and any structures in their way. When a person falls, the direction they fall in will vary according to many factors; the complexity can be as extreme as the seemingly endless and variable divisions of these tree branches.*

One cannot always separate falls into distinct groups, because they can, of course, be a mixture, some being extremely complex. In addition, with each type of fall, just like the branching of a tree, there are endless directions, as well as angles, in which you can fall. The complex branching of a willow tree is shown (see photograph 3-d) to remind us of how complex a fall can be.

When you fall, the drop is not always simply backward, sideways or forward. It can be complicated by a downward rotation. In other words, many falls are made worse by people *rotating* down at various angles, with various parts of the body projected in different directions, and striking any variety of objects on the ground as they approach the surface they are falling toward.

Now add to this complex mixture another important ingredient.

If the person falling is stiff with arthritis, is feeling frozen because of cold weather, or is just not concentrating on what is happening around them for any reason, and particularly if they are unskilled in landing methods, it could well be the head that hits the ground first. From this example, you can see that, if all conditions are right when falling, a fall injury can be simple and painless, but it can be complex and deadly if you fall in a 'bad' way.

Please study the five chapters 16 to 20 that show how to avoid the 'bad' way to fall.

Drowning occurs if you have an accident in water, and falling injuries occur if you have an accident on land or some other solid surface. So, learn to *swim* to reduce your risks of drowning, and learn to *land skillfully* to reduce your risk of experiencing one or more of the many nasty injuries that can result from a fall. Fortunately, suffering one of the many injuries described above does not always kill you. Many who suffer a fracture, even doctors, are surprised at how painful it can be. In fact, doctors who suffer fractures are the most surprised of all! Most fracture pains are severe, and some of the strongest painkillers ever designed are needed to provide comfort to the victim of the injury.

Now, let us get back to the money talk. What is your most valuable possession? Is it your house, your car, or perhaps an antique violin? Whatever it is, people tend to treat their most valuable possession with the greatest respect, for example, a person with a new car drives and parks it with great care. If you had to carry an antique vase down a stairway, or from one place to another, you would grip it firmly and walk carefully, and then place it down gently to avoid damage. *If* we were to be as careful with our *bodies* as we are with our various precious items, we would probably never get hurt from an injury.

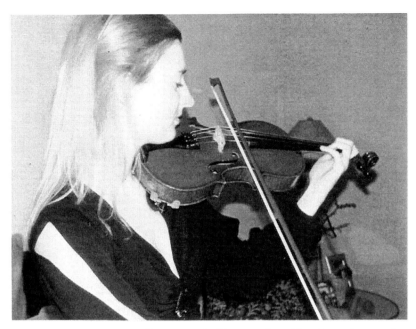

3-e   Monica's violin is one of her most valuable possessions. There is one item worth a lot more to her and her family. Do you know what that is?

Photograph 3-e shows Monica, a talented violinist, rehearsing for a concert. This wonderful musician loves her violin, but she regards *her body and her looks* as considerably more valuable than any of the world's most famous musical instruments. Monica practises so that she can perfect her recital or performance. In our daily lives, as well, practice makes perfect in any skills training, and this includes balance, Ground Reflex and Landing Skills (GRALS — more of which later), muscle toning, posture, and every other action that improves or maintains good health.

What I am really trying to say here is this:

Our most valuable possession — always and forever — is our body!

Yes, everything from the hair or skin on the outside to the structures on the inside, which of course includes our brains, our muscles, our bones, our blood, and every single tissue, has to be treated with the greatest respect.

The seven bars of soap shown in photograph 3-f are not here to test your recognition skills. For example, they could represent a close-up photograph of a pile of seven white tablets. This soap could also be a reminder to wash your hands before and after handling food or using the wash-room. Really, though, it is related to our topic of the value of our bodies, and our next comment is morbid but true.

Do you want to know some more *facts* about what the human body is worth?

Fact 1: The value of the chemicals in the body of an average human being is not much. I have seen estimates that vary from about $2 (£1 sterling) to $5 (£2 sterling)!

Fact 2: An average human being has enough meat on them to serve 75 meals at one sitting!

Fact 3: An average human being has enough fat on them to make seven bars of soap!

Our body, of course, is worth far more than 75 meals and seven bars of soap!

3-f Seven bars of soap

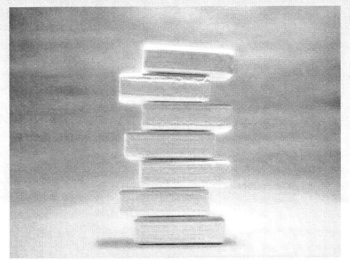

There are endless ways in which our precious tissues can be damaged or destroyed, as can be seen from the "injury tree."

Now, let us look at the parts of our body that can be injured, and what those injuries could be. All injuries can be serious, even a simple scratch, for example, can open a way for the flesh-eating bug to enter our bodies. When hiking on long trails, a small knee graze can develop into a larger patch of inflamed skin because of the effects of friction caused by clothing material. As a result of an increasingly painful knee wound, the ability to lift the foot will be reduced, thus increasing the chance of a major fall. This book, however, is designed to prevent head and other more dangerous types of trauma caused by falls, but one can also minimize even slight injuries by practising what this book offers. Diagram 3-g shows not only a rather fit-looking woman just raring to go but also the parts of the body that suffer when one experiences a fall of any type.

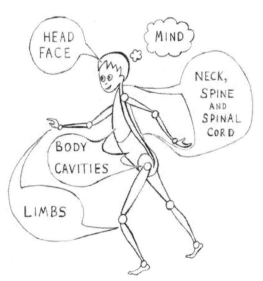

3-g The injury zones of the body

3-g The Injury Points and Protection Zones that You Need
To Know when Landing from a Fall

Some injuries that are possible:

Fractures and/or dislocations

Soft tissue injuries to the tendons and ligaments

skin, face, eyes and ears

muscles

brain, spinal cord and

nerves

blood vessels

internal organs (liver, spleen,

kidneys, heart, lungs, etc)

Psychological/Psychiatric disorders

Note that, even if you avoid a fracture, psychological suffering, including becoming *fearful of falling* (as well as colliding with a surface), can often result from this type of trauma (this fear is described below).

"Things" that We Hate To Hear About in the World of Falling Trauma

Nasty injuries that can occur in the areas of the body shown on our athletic woman are as follows:

Head   Brain damage, skull fractures and scalp tears, with lots of complications.

Face   Cuts leading to scars, nose damage with possibly visible distortion, fractures of the cheeks, the zygomatics, and other face bones, including the teeth and the jaws. One is hesitant to mention it, but the eyes can be punctured and the ear lobes can be ripped as well.

Neck, spine and spinal cord   Dislocations and fractures, along with severe muscle tendon strains, can, of course, occur in this part of the body with many types of falls. Classes of injury such as motor vehicle collisions are other ways that this part of the body can be damaged. Spinal cord damage can be caused by neck and spine trauma, resulting in varying degrees of paralysis.

Body cavities   The three main body cavities are shown in our athletic woman.

Chest — The ribs, the lungs and the heart are the more serious structures likely to suffer in this most important zone. On the surface of this cavity are, of course, the breasts, and these can be injured as easily as any other surface protrusion. Even those women who have had both breasts removed because of cancer in this region are vulnerable to scar tissue damage on the chest wall.

Breast implants can rupture with or without an impacting force, leading to the many possible complications caused by leaking material that is foreign to human body tissues.

Abdominal — Major organs, such as the liver, the kidneys, the spleen, the pancreas, and the intestine, are all at risk to a large number of types of damage when falling, especially onto protruding objects.

Pelvic — If one is unlucky enough to fall from a height, or even just from a standing position, onto a sharp object, there is a chance that a puncture through to the pelvic organs could occur. The rectum, the vagina, the urethra, and the bladder can be torn severely, resulting in permanent internal scarring.

Limbs Broken bones, torn ligaments and tendons, sprains, damaged cartilage, and dislocations, all along with skin tears, are possible with any type of fall.

The fear of falling, along with the depression caused by any disability or cosmetic change that results from body damage, cannot be ignored.

Basophobia is the term used for an extreme fear of falling from either a standing position or a walking activity. Other phobias that can develop are fears of accidents generally (*dystychiphobia* or *traumatophobia*) and of falling down stairs (*climacophobia*).

"I feel really embarrassed and stupid." This comment is uttered by many people after they have had a fall, even when they are seriously injured. This self-inflicted humiliation can be avoided if and when you fall simply by landing in a skillful manner.

Because these psychological conditions are quite common, at any age, and following any type of collision with any surface below us, landing in a *good* way should be our goal *when* we fall.

Thus, knowledge of the injury zones is a useful way to understand the danger points of the body, that is, those parts of the body that are at risk of damage from various types of fall. Please get to know these zones well, and develop a strategy, with the help of the information provided in the *5x5 Mix* chapters, to not allow these body zones to be hurt in any way or *to at least reduce the severity* of the trauma that is possible from taking a tumble.

Chapter 4

'Tunnel' Everything

An organ to be treasured, especially when it is working well, is that 'jewel' of special senses and many colors — the eye. The majority of us value our good vision, and I am sure that most of us appreciate this special sense even more when we see those who are unfortunate enough to be blind or to have poor eyesight.

There are strict standards in most countries to regulate the operation of a motor vehicle. One of these standards is to ensure that all adults have acceptable vision to be able to drive a car, a truck or a motorcycle.

Despite their good vision, many vehicle drivers describe incidents where they have collided with another vehicle/object/person but deny having seen anything in their way! Other situations, not involving collisions, have also been described, such as people who have driven illegally through a red light at a road junction, insisting that they did not see it! Then there are cases of people who, after driving long distances, arrive at their destinations without any memory of the journey, often claiming that they did not see anything on the way!

People interested in our failure to use our perfectly good eyes to see what is happening around us have performed studies. One such study, designed by a television news team, took an unusually dressed-up person and had them walk alongside busy traffic while a television reporter randomly stopped vehicles to check which drivers had seen the out-of-place character. Amazingly, and despite that the oddly dressed-up character was actually on the road surface, often within a few feet of the drivers, most of those drivers did not notice anything at all!

In the above situations, the drivers were not blindfolded, but obviously something was affecting their ability to use their eyesight effectively. What was that something?

We have all heard of tunnel vision. This term is usually applied to people who suffer from certain eye diseases, or occasionally disorders of the brain, that affect what is called their *fields of vision*. These people can see objects that they look straight at, but while looking at that object everything around it is not seen — it is as if one is looking at that object through a narrow cardboard tube with one eye.

Anyone who has experienced tunnel vision, or has been told that they could have it, or something like it, for example, walking into objects frequently and driving through a red light at a road intersection, should have thorough eye and nervous system examinations.

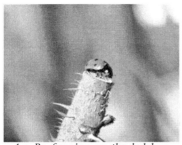

4-a By focusing on the ladybug, everything around is blurred

Photograph 4-a shows what we are talking about, in that the center of the photograph is in focus, whereas the outer portion is not. We can call this outer portion the peripheral zone, and use our *surround vision* to make us aware of the objects in this fuzzy region. (Photograph 4-a shows a focused ladybug with a blurred background, and photograph 4-b shows a focused car with a blurred rock in the foreground.)

Just as our central vision is important, so is our surround

4-b As you focus on the car, the rock's distinct outline is diminished

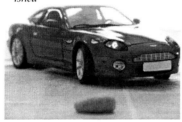

vision. As we gaze ahead, we should see not only the area that we are focusing on but also the large zones around that area.

There are various ways in which there could be a distortion in these so-called fields of vision. They can be divided into four major groups as follows:

Surround Vision Interference — Four Major Causes

Medical Reasons	
Direct	glaucoma, disease of the retina, eyelid sagging, brain tumors
Non-direct	pain anywhere, neck stiffness

Obstructed	
Accidental	direct sunlight reflection, objects in the way, rain
Built-in	carrying objects (eg, a tray), wearing a hat, in-car obstructions (poor design or objects blocking the view)

Distractions	
Inner	depression, worrying, anxiety, and many other similar situations
Outer	mobile/cellular telephones, interactions with other people or animals, noise (radio, etc), and other distractions

Surround Vision Interference   Four Major Causes (Con't)

Apparent

Camouflaged variety of dangers car same color as background, dark objects in shadows, flashing lights/signs, and many others

A cat blends in with the background and feels quite safe from a local coyote who will not be able to see her as long as she keeps still. This is a good example of camouflage, but in the lives of humans we hope that we will notice camouflaged dangers. (photograph 4-c).

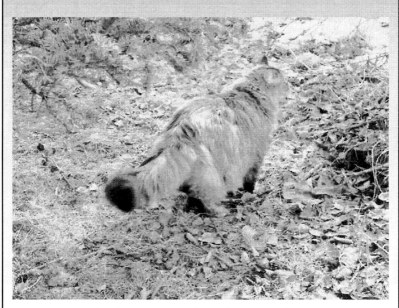

4-c An example of a camouflaged cat. Sometimes dangers are hidden because they blend in with their background.

The summer cartoon depicted below is an attempt to show some of the ways that surround vision is reduced (even in people without a medical problem). Cartoon 4-d is a disaster about to happen, so read on to see why.

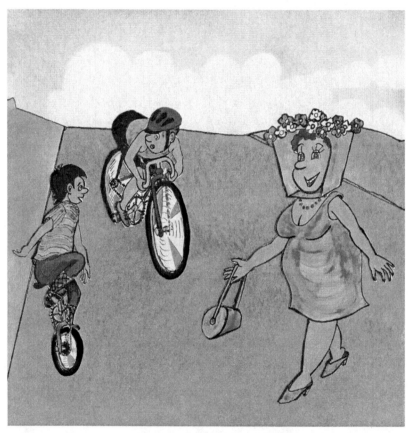

4-d All three people are about to suffer preventable injuries

Ms Freddi is busy thinking about her determined effort to reduce her body weight; she has decided to walk to the shops to buy some lemons. Extremely conscious of her looks, she has been reading the fashion and health maga-

zines, which tell her that too much sun can cause skin cancer. The fancy hat that she is wearing shades her face well,
and at the same time the flowers have been added to keep
her attractive (she saw this in her fashion magazine as
well).

In the meantime, over the hill comes a speedy cyclist, who
notes 'competition' in the form of a child practising spins
on his unicycle. The child not wearing a helmet turns in
the excitement of seeing the approaching cyclist.

This is a bad situation! Ms Freddi's surround vision is ob-
structed by her hat, as well she is busy thinking about her
shopping and her health. In fact, she is probably not seeing
much at all! In the meantime, the speeding cyclist has been
distracted by a 'one-wheeled wonder,' who in turn is distracted by the cyclist. At the least, Ms Freddi and the cyclist
are doomed for an injury. The result of the collision could
cause the child to fall. To make matters worse, the hel-
metless child in this cartoon is vulnerable to a head injury,
which could maim or even kill him.

Need I say more!

In any injury situation, *using your eyes to the maximum* can
help to lessen the risk of serious damage, or in some cases
even prevent the injury. One would think that it should be

a natural skill to use our surround vision (perhaps it was at one time, many years ago in the evolutionary process), but for whatever variety of reasons many people do not use it efficiently.

Is there a way to improve the situation?

It might not be possible to use our surround vision continually during our waking hours; however, if each person interested in reducing injuries, which should be everyone, is aware of all situations where body damage can occur and is able to switch on their direct + surround vision at those critical moments when an injury is most likely to happen, this should help to reduce considerably the damage to your most valuable possession   your body! Using this sense, you could also help to reduce injury to those people who happen to be with or near you; *you* can be *their* eyes.

Binocular vision is another important sense that we have as humans, as long as we can use *both* our eyes. When looking at something, each eye sees that same object at a slightly different angle, and as a result of this slightly different view the retina sees two slightly different images, thus creating the sense of *depth or distance*. If you can only use one eye, then you cannot usually judge distance! A device that shows this effect well, and which many children love as a toy, is the stereoscope. When the pictures that fit into the device are examined, two images are seen of the same scene. Each image is slightly different, so that, when viewed in the stereoscope, a three-dimensional image is seen. To be able to judge distance is obviously an important sense to have working well; however, for people who have only one eye that works well, it is possible to train that single eye and the brain to judge distance. With help and practice, along with logic, a sense of distance can be relearned. A simple example of the logic method is that, by knowing the size of a variety of other objects, you can compare them with the environment that you are in. So, if you are in a town with people and traffic around, knowing the size of cars, the height of people, the spacing of lamp-posts, etc, you can compare those items, thereby using them to help you to judge distance.

Training is necessary to improve the efficiency of your eyes/vision. It is this training, along with the practice of other rules of body injury prevention, that can prevent or reduce the seriousness of trauma.

As children, we should all remember being told, time and time again, that before crossing the road we should look "left, right, and then left again," or "right, left, and then right again," depending upon which country you grew up in. This drill was, of course, designed to brainwash us as children to watch out for traffic and to avoid getting hit, that is, to avoid an injury.

Every day, it is sad to see many adults walk onto a busy road without any attempt to look for the danger of a car or truck heading their way. These often intelligent people seem to think that a heavy, moving vehicle can just stop suddenly, just because they want to cross the road when they feel like doing so. This type of injury or even death should never happen. It seems from observations and opinions that the kind of people who regularly walk across a busy road, without even so much as a glance to see if there is traffic, feel that the law allows them to act as if they were blind. Laws do protect pedestrians, but those 'secure people' could end up dead or paralyzed if they happen to be hit by a vehicle; no lawyer can take that away!

Injuries do not always come from one direction. What is meant by this is that your *awareness* should not be just *ahead* of you. Just because you are looking forward does not mean that you are aware of what is going on *around* you. You have to be able to be aware of what is *below* you, what is *above* you, what is to the *left* and *right* of your body, and what is *behind* you. One good habit to develop is that while you are looking ahead try to be aware of what is above, below, and to the left or right of you — all at the same time! This is truly using your surround vision and should become a habit.

Unfortunately, we do not have eyes in the back of our heads, so developing being aware of what is behind us is quite an acquired art. Without being paranoid, and by using all your senses, including your memory, ways can be developed to help you to be aware of what is behind you. Of course, if you are in your car, you can use your rearview or side mirrors to observe what is behind you, but if you are just out for a walk, you have to use, from the minute you leave your home or car, your hearing, your smell, and your vision, and occasionally you should stop to look around you, just to be aware of any nearby dangers.

Dangers from Various Directions

Here are some injuries that can occur from any variety of angle from your body 'sphere.'

From Above   Objects falling from houses or other buildings, fruit or branches from trees, projectiles from upper levels in shopping malls, and from the sky (debris blown by the wind, attacking birds, hornets or killer bee hives, etc). Photograph 4-e shows a wasp nest just overhead.

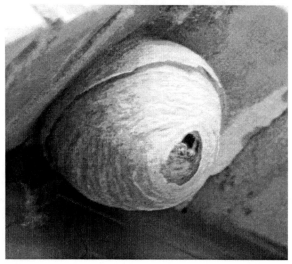

4-e Wasp nests such as this one can be just above your head

From Below   Materials on the ground (blunt objects, sharp glass and wire, animal traps, etc), manholes/holes/openings in the ground/floor, snakes, sheer drops or other sudden level changes. Photographs 4-f and 4-g show gopher holes, and *4–h* shows a small but live snake. Barbed wire can be a hazard both to trip over and to land on. Photograph *4 -i* shows loops of barbed wire broken away from a post. It can be hidden in shadows or in the snow, and it can become almost invisible at night.

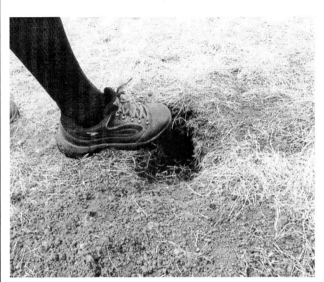

4-f A gopher hole is usually just big enough for a foot to slip into

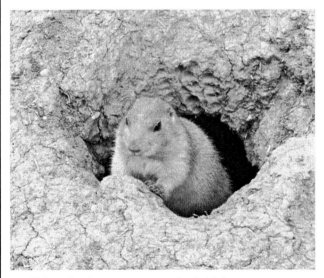

4-g This gopher does not want your foot in his home

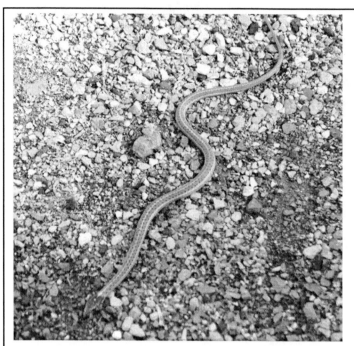

4-h It is surprising what you will see if you keep your eyes on the ground

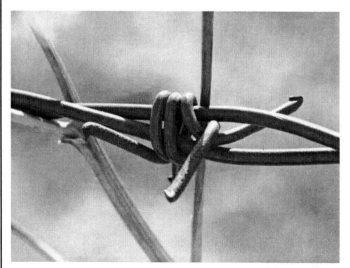

4-i Barbed wire is a ground level hazard and easy to trip on

From Behind   This includes many of the above, especially if you are walking backward (see photograph 4-j). Intentional injuries are common here too. And when on the beach, with your back to the ocean, beware of sneaker waves because they can be extremely powerful and drag you into the depths of the water in an instant! Photograph *4-k* shows approaching waves that are extremely power-ful, and so, if you are relaxing on a beach, this potentially deadly force has to be taken seriously.

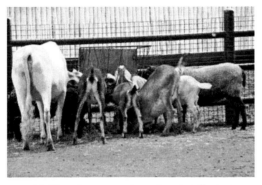

4-j These hungry creatures do not really care what or who is behind them, but you should!

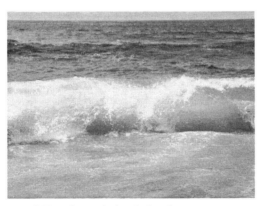

4-k Have fun at the beach, but do not turn your back on the ocean for long

> *From the Side*   There are many examples of course, left or right: vehicles and moving objects, intentional attacks by people or animals, flames, fires, electrical, ledges that you can fall from, as well as other objects that can be tripped over, or that can hit you.

To summarize so far, whether at home, at work, driving or just going for a walk, allow your surround vision to be switched on, using head or body rotation, so that you can see in as many directions as possible. Regularly direct your vision behind you, so that you can survey your surroundings more fully.

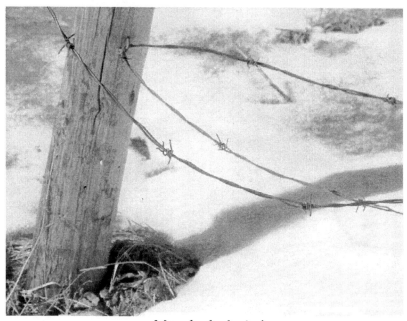

More barbed wire!

The *body sphere* referred to above is equivalent to your personal space in meaning. This topic is also dealt with in the chapter on posture. It refers to an imaginary space around a person's body, and for convenience it is divided into different levels, where the distances vary according to the person's personality and cultural background. If you like, they can be called comfort regions, and they are usually divided into five sections.

1) Closest to the body is the *Touching Region* (up to 6 inches)

2) The *One-foot Length Region* (6 to 18 inches from the body surface)

3) The *One-to-two Arms, Length Region* (about 20 to 40 inches from the body surface)

4) The *Room-sized (Social) Region* (up to 10 feet away)

5) The *Outdoor* or *Public Region* (over 10 feet away)

These regions are important, in that any undesirable object or living being entering the wrong region at the wrong time could be a psychological or physical risk to you.

What is extremely important is that you do not treat familiar surroundings, such as your home or neighborhood, as necessarily safe. Out of habit, we tend to move about our homes casually, assuming in our minds that the floor and surroundings are in the same state that they were seconds, minutes or hours before. An example of this is that you might be walking downstairs in the dark. Because these stairs were clear of objects the day before, in your mind you feel that the stairs will still be clear of such objects. Unbeknown to you, however, someone might have had a paint can on the stairs since then and forgotten to remove it. The result of this could potentially be a disaster, as shown in cartoon 4-1!

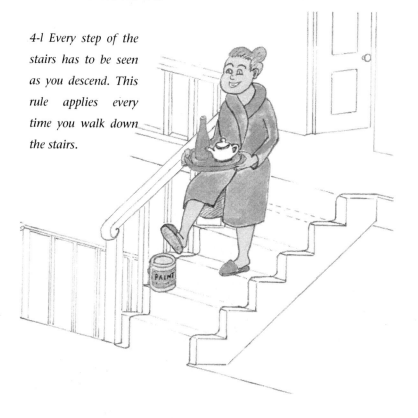

4-1 Every step of the stairs has to be seen as you descend. This rule applies every time you walk down the stairs.

Many motor vehicle injuries occur when the driver is in a familiar environment. As a result perhaps of fatigue and the dropping of one's guard, many people are maimed or killed close to home. So, as you get close to your home territory, raise your determination to complete the trip without an accident, and practise surround thinking even as you enter your dwelling place.

To paraphrase a well-known saying, "Familiarity can breed injuries!" unless you stop yourself from developing bad habits now. So, without making yourself excessively nervous, always expect the unexpected.

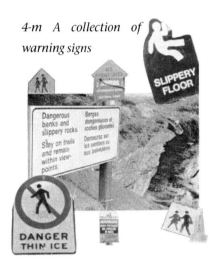

4-m A collection of warning signs

At this point, again, remember that *most accidents occur within or close to your own home!*

There are not enough signs around to help remind us from one minute to the next of how to avoid falling injuries, or in fact any type of injury. The collection of signs shown in photograph 4-m are not enough to impact the seriously high incidence of fall-type injuries. A sign, such as the one shown here (photograph 4-n) warning you of sea lions, would make anyone extra-alert, so try to be aware of the dangers around you without a need for signs. Keep in mind that, unless you

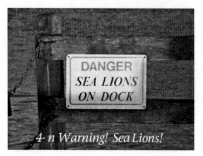

4- n Warning! Sea Lions!

provide them, there will be no warnings in and around your home!

Referring back to the title of this chapter, I should now define the term 'tunnel' everything. It means not only tunnel vision but also tunnel thinking, tunnel hearing and tunnel mentality. It means, whether at home or away from home, that *we have to keep our vision and minds open in all directions!*

Thinking of the wrong thing at the wrong time can lead to injuries. So, here are some repeat statements because they are worth repeating.

If you can *perfect your vision,* as mentioned above; *sharpen your awareness* of how injuries occur and how you can prevent them; *perfect your balance,* and your *knowledge and skills in landing* from a fall; *strengthen* the weak points of your body, keep your body tissues *healthy* with correct nutrition and exercise, and maintain a *perfect posture,* then you are well on your way to being able to prevent one of the most serious diseases that affects humankind.

Chapter 5

Human Landing Gear

Imagine that you are standing on a chair to reach for something that you need. You fall because the chair slips away, but you land in such a way that you are able to get up immediately, finding that you are not hurt at all! Whether it be falling from a high point such as a chair or slipping on ice, landing on the ground and not getting hurt, even though it sounds as if you are an indestructible character in a cartoon situation, *is actually possible in real life!*

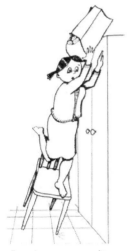

5-a A common situation for a fall in the kitchen. Is a limb fracture or head injury inevitable?

As already mentioned, a common fall in the home is a drop down to the floor off a chair in the kitchen. Our injury prone character (see cartoon 5-a) is reaching for stored cans of food and using a chair to raise herself up. The chair legs slide out from under her; there is no doubt where she is about to go. This is our reminder that falls in the home are extremely common, especially in the kitchen, in the bathroom, and on stairs.

No matter how much you know about *avoiding* falls, you will at some time fall, but it is hoped that you will not get hurt.

So, if life were perfect, you would either not fall at all or, if you did fall, you would land in such a way that you would not break bones or experience any other injuries. In fact, falling over would not be such a bad thing at all. We are born with neither flippers nor fins, but we can still learn to swim in water, for safety, for fun and for sport.

We human beings have learned to travel in a variety of environments that we were not necessarily designed for and that we are not really meant to be in. If one considers pastimes or sports such as skydiving, using parachutes to land safely on the ground; or learning to travel on ice, using ice skates; or on snow, using skis, they show how we can adapt well to seemingly unnatural activities. These activities use specialized equipment to enable a person to participate, but one has to learn the skills necessary to be able to use the devices for the activity, whether it be for fun, for sport or for work. Aerial skiing, for instance, is a great example of the human ability to be able to perform many complex spins and rotations in the air and land upright on the ground. Despite spinning high in the air, the aerial skier (see illustration 5-b) can watch the horizon, rotate the body, and land smoothly on the snow, on skis, and without falling over.

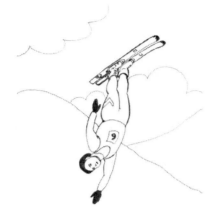

5-b If human beings can land on their feet from this aerial ski position, then most people should be able to learn to land on the ground in a safe way from a simple fall!

What is the similarity between an airplane and a human being? The answer to this question is simple. If either of these 'bodies' *leaves/takes off* from the ground surface, it has to land again eventually. When airplanes land on the ground, it has to be done as smoothly as possible for the comfort and safety of the passengers. To land in this way, preferably the airplane has to be structurally sound with good working parts. The pilot has to be trained and in good working order as well. Making contact with the ground is made possible with landing gear. In the case of an airplane landing on solid ground, the landing gear used consists of wheels with tires and shock absorbers.

If human beings were fitted with landing gear, and our structures were always tough, when we took off — as in a fall — we could also land just like an airplane, smoothly and safely. But because we are not born with obvious landing gear to land safely from a fall, it is possible to develop parts of our bodies to behave just like landing gear. The question is: How do we do this?

Training your body to land safely like an airplane is not done by using any of the regular exercises that the average person is trained in, but by learning the skills that enable you to land from a fall in such a way that you can reduce the shock to your body as it hits the ground. Without discussing the laws of physics that govern this, what you do is either spread the impact forces, so that the shock does not concentrate on one point of the body, or deflect the forces of the impact by hitting the ground in a circular fashion — just like a rolling ball. Along with learning the skills to guide your body to direct itself safely in a fall, parts of your body can be trained to act just like shock absorbers.

So far, the above activity sounds complicated; however, as soon as you are introduced to additional details of this ideal plan in the landing skills chapter, this and other important ways to reduce injuries will make "human landing gear" more understandable.

Let us look at some examples from the animal kingdom. Seals and otters have the perfect design for swimming, but apart from using their flippers or feet for directing their flow through the water they can also use all four flippers for walking on solid ground. Humans, however, are designed for walking on solid ground, but we have learned to use our limbs to swim either for safety or fun. The otter shown here (see photograph 5-c) is in "land mode."

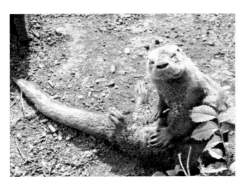

5--c *This curious otter's ability to use its limbs for walking, running and swimming is well-known*

A simple drawing (see illustration 5-d) shows a human swimming with some seals: the latter being the more efficient movers in water, but not as quick on land. As suggested above, both can adapt to the two different environments.

Keeping with the animal kingdom, because we humans can learn so much from animal survival skills, one of the most superbly designed creatures on this planet is the cat (photograph 5-e). This stealthy animal, whether large or small, has some enviable features. Cats are extremely flexible, and they have superb reflexes and excellent vision (both day and night), along with tremendous hearing and a heightened sense of smell. I am particularly interested in

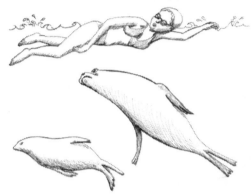

5-d This woman's arms and legs can be trained for swimming, and in seals, who can naturally swim, the flippers can also be used for walking

the so-called "nine lives" that a cat apparently has; moreover, as children, we learn that a cat can jump, fall or be dropped from great heights without apparent injury. Published studies, such as those reported in the *Journal of the American Veterinary Medical Association* (Dr. G. Robinson, 1976; and Whitney, W., and Mehlhaff, C., 1987), have documented cases where cats have dropped or fallen from buildings on average more than five stories and have survived the fall 90% of the time. In fact, the record height for a cat surviving a fall is an astounding 45 stories high — not bad for a mammal without wings!

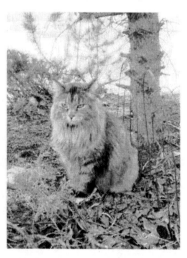

5-e The cat is an expert at landing from great heights using its limbs to absorb the shock of impact with the ground

Research is continuing in an attempt to try to discover the secret of the cat's ability to fall and land without injury. The answer to this fall injury resistance will likely be found in the design of the cat's bones, muscles and tendons, along with the balance and reflex abilities of this springy creature (see the chapters on osteoporosis for more interesting cat information).

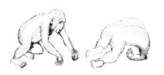

5-f Chimpanzees, especially in play, roll forward. They are not taught to roll there body but do so instinctively and quite freely and naturally, seemingly having fun with this action. Human beings can be shown how to roll the same way as chimpanzees for exercise, for safety in accidental falls, and just for fun.

Another interesting group of animals are the ape family. Most species of apes and monkeys are also, like the cat, extremely flexible. I am sure that many people have noted this from the behavior of these often noisy, playful animals, who can jump from branch to branch in trees, drop to the ground with ease, roll freely on the ground, and seem to have fun doing so. The chimpanzee diagrams (see illustration 5-f) reveal the ways in which these powerful animals can roll, as well as rotate their bodies, while running. The exercise portion of this book, moreover, reveals how humans can also learn to perform these chimpanzee activities for the development of fitness and safety skills, and for sheer fun.

So, let us summarize our ideas so far. *If we could land like an airplane, fall like a cat, and roll like a chimpanzee,* falling would cause nowhere near as many injuries as are seen at present, which is a time when these injuries are actually increasing. Airplanes can of course crash for a large variety of reasons, and in the same way we cannot land perfectly every time, but if we have the skills and make an effort to use them we do stand a good chance of meeting the ground safely!

Those readers who have disabilities or who suffer other forms of ill health, including painful conditions, are often at a higher risk of a fall injury, and although this particular information is not specializing in activities for people with a physical handicap many of the skills shown in the exercise chapters can be practised.

It is well-known that physical activity and training in any exercise system present many barriers to patients, whether they come from being excessively overweight, from experiencing persistent tiredness, or from suffering from one of the common ailments, such as arthritis, or one of the many other disabling illnesses.

In Chapters 16 to 20, even if you suffer disorders of the back or the knees, most of the warm-up exercises should be possible.

For the strengthening activities, avoid the sit-up type of exercise if you suffer a low back disorder, and avoid the forward and lateral spinal flexion in the stretching section.

If you suffer from a knee disorder, then you should avoid the knee walking and crawling techniques listed in Chapter 19.

Chapter 20 demonstrates the basic home version of landing skills. The short list that follows advises which skills to avoid for some common medical problems.

Low back disorders: Care should be taken with skills B, C and perhaps E, and K.
Knee disorders: Care should be taken with skills C, D, F, I and perhaps K.
Wrist and shoulder: Take care with the force of striking the mat surface. Even if you tap the mat surface only gently, you will at least develop a reflex in landing ability.

Remember this point. If you do have a wrist, shoulder, knee or back disorder, think what would happen if you

fell and hit the ground with a heavy blow and had neither the landing skills nor the ability to prevent the fall!

Even if you suffer pain, it is worth the effort to achieve
a higher level of fitness, and if possible to develop skills
in landing in a safe way. Common sense will help you
to decide which exercises you can or cannot do. If you
are not sure, ask your health adviser.

Although it is not an encyclopedia on medical disorders, Chapter 12 does describe some common physical
complaints, as do the chapters on perimenopause. Many
of these medical problems carry an inherent risk of falling over.

It is not suggested here that you grow wings, but simply
that you try to develop efficient landing gear.
So, if you fall down, it is hoped that you have a happy
landing!

Chapter 6

The Story of Osteoporosis — Part One —
How You Get Weak Bones

Once upon a time, the word "osteoporosis" was not written in any book, but around the mid-1940s it did start to appear in medical articles and journals. Health practitioners have recognized for centuries that some groups of people, including children, are prone to breaking bones. Old books on health, from one hundred years ago for example, frequently mention that old age is associated with a higher risk of breaking bones. These same health advisory texts describe diet and exercise as important parts of one's lifestyle, and suggest that milk should be an important part of one's diet, but they do not say why these recommendations are necessary. One author advises, in a chapter on old age, that violent exercise should be avoided because it can break bones, but the wording only implies that with advanced years bones are more fragile, and a name for those weakened bones is not given. Having said this, it should be pointed out that bone architecture was first shown to be affected by the loads applied to it more than three hundred years ago by the celebrated Italian scientist Galileo Galilei.

Since Galileo's time, other scientists have been interested in the way that bone is affected by age and diet, along with the mechanics of bone strength. Once osteoporosis was described by medical scientists and recognised as a disease, the research expanded, a prevention approach was developed, and treatments were found to treat people both old and young. Thus, as indicated in the previous statement, osteoporosis is not just a disease of old age.

Present-day important *facts:*

Osteoporosis is a disease of bone

Osteoporosis makes bones weaker than healthy bone

Osteoporosis causes bones to break more easily

Broken bones can maim you!

Broken bones (fractures) can kill you!

Osteoporosis, therefore, can kill as well as disable people.

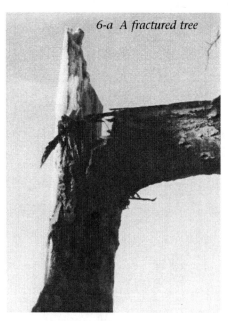

6-a A fractured tree

Photograph 6-a shows a relatively young tree that has been broken, snapped by the wind, and it has sustained damage that is impossible to repair. A bone breaks in a similar manner to a tree trunk, but it is repairable, and is in many cases even preventable.

So what is all the fuss about osteoporosis in the

last decade or so? You hear a lot about this bone disease now for at least three reasons:

1) Tests of various types can diagnose osteoporosis.

2) Continually improving treatments are now available for osteoporosis.

3) People are living longer, and age, although it is not the only factor that causes osteoporosis, is one of the primary reasons for it. So, because there are more old people, this disease is more common.

Did you know that a bone is not just a collection of crystals and protein? Like other tissues of the body, bone is similar to a city, in that the structures and population are constantly flowing. The hive of activity or city-like business in living bone, with its continual traffic of cells and chemicals, and the buildup of structures, as well as their demolition, are controlled by many factors. Hormones, nutrition, and stresses and strains acting upon the architecture, as well as chemicals in the bloodstream, all have a powerful influence on the health or prosperity of living bone.

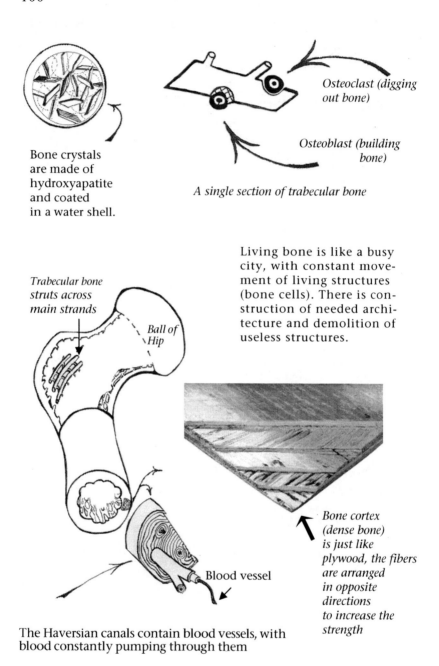

Bone crystals
are made of
hydroxyapatite
and coated
in a water shell.

*Osteoclast (digging
out bone)*

*Osteoblast (building
bone)*

A single section of trabecular bone

*Trabecular bone
struts across
main strands*

*Ball of
Hip*

Living bone is like a busy
city, with constant move-
ment of living structures
(bone cells). There is con-
struction of needed architecture and demolition of
useless structures.

*Bone cortex
(dense bone)
is just like
plywood, the fibers
are arranged
in opposite
directions
to increase the
strength*

Blood vessel

The Haversian canals contain blood vessels, with
blood constantly pumping through them

6-b Bone anatomy

Osteoid is bone without the crystals. Another name for this osteoid is bone matrix, and it is mostly made of collagen (about 30% of bone is the matrix).

Trabecular bone is also called cancellous (spongy or lattice-like) bone. It looks porous, and the strands are arranged to withstand forces such as compression, as well as pulling. Again, the main strands are braced to increase the strength.

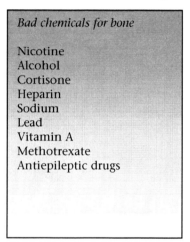

Good chemicals for bone	Bad chemicals for bone
Vitamin D	Nicotine
Parathormone	Alcohol
Phosphorus	Cortisone
Magnesium	Heparin
Vitamin C	Sodium
Testosterone	Lead
Fluoride	Vitamin A
Carbonates	Methotrexate
Estrogen	Antiepileptic drugs
Calcium	
Citrates	
Calcitonin	
Osteopontin	

The chemicals mentioned above can be both good or bad for bone function and structure: good chemicals can help bone tissues become stronger, whereas bad chemicals can make bones weaker.

Please see photograph/diagram 6-b, which illustrates what bone is made of and why it is so strong, at least when all the bone ingredients are present and arranged in a correct way to withstand the variety of forces that are exerted upon them.

Do you know this medical condition? Osteopenia is the name used to describe when bone density is low, but not low enough to be called osteoporosis.

Another fact that is not appreciated is that osteoporosis does not have to be in every bone in the body. For example, it might be present in the hip or in the spine but not in the lower bones of the leg. The parts of the body that are tested the most are the backbone (spine), the hips and the wrists; however, if even just one bone is weaker than normal, then that same person is at risk of osteopenia or osteoporosis in other bones as well.

As suggested above, osteoporosis creates fragile bone because the internal parts of the structure are weakened by a thinning-out process of important weight-bearing regions. Even if people look healthy on the outside, their bones can be diseased, just as if those structures were aging quicker than the rest of the body. Photograph 6-c shows an extremely porous-looking tree; it is weak and prone to breaking easily — a lot like osteoporotic bone! In the information below,

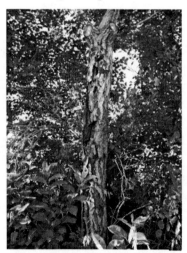

6-c A porous tree trunk

various bone cells are described, of which two are important in the process of osteoporosis. *Osteoblasts* help to make new bone; *osteoclasts* can destroy it. So, if *osteoclasts* eat bone away quicker than the *osteoblasts* can make it, on average there is a bone loss from the body. If loss of bone occurs, the skeleton is made weaker, and so it is easier for fractures to occur. This, then, is the basis for osteoporosis. The secret to the strength and lightness of bone lies in its anatomy, in chemical content, and in its surrounding supporting structures. Let us now look at these three important features of bone strength.

Bone Anatomy   Refer to diagram/photograph 6-b, where it is noted that bone has a surrounding, dense cortex made up of layers or sheets of leathery collagen, which is packed with needlelike crystals of a chemical called hydroxyapatite. This chemical is made up, of course, of calcium and phosphorus, elements essential to bone for its toughness in resisting compression, that is, the forces that squash down on your body.

Scientists consider bone to be made of an organic matrix (the collagen/protein portion of bone) and the mineral matrix (the crystal portion — calcium, phosphorus and some other minerals, such as magnesium).

Included in this bone anatomy are the blood vessels and three types of cell: the osteocyte (a type of stationary or trapped osteoblast), the active osteoblast and the osteoclast.

Bone *cortex* is made up of tightly packed alternating layers of bone (much like plywood, see diagram/photograph 6-b). In certain areas of bones that take a lot of weight, the internal bone, that is, the bone that is not in the cortex (see diagram/photograph 6-b), is arranged in strands called *trabeculae*. These trabeculae act like the trusses in a bridge structure, adding superior strength, but without lots of weight.

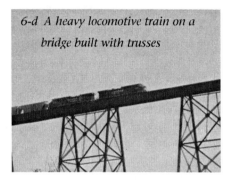

6-d *A heavy locomotive train on a bridge built with trusses*

If you look at photograph 6-d, the bridge has to support an extremely heavy, moving locomotive train, which it does with ease because of the cross braces that are holding the upright posts. In osteoporosis, the bone trabeculae thin out quicker than the rest of the bone because of its higher metabolism, thereby reducing bone weight/density, and thus bone strength.

One of the most important qualities of bone is its flexibility, because hardness in itself is not enough to resist a fracture, especially when a long bone is stressed in a bending fashion. To be flexible, the bone collagen has to be of good quality, and the cross braces of the trabeculae have to be intact, with full mineral content.

Refer back to diagram/photograph 6-b now for a summary of its meanings. Living, *healthy* bone is just like a bustling major city — when it has a healthy budget!

Bone, on the outside, looks fairly quiet and inactive to the average person's eye, but under the microscope there is a totally different picture. Instead of people standing and moving, there are the various bone cells, in the millions, constantly working, or at least ready for action. These bone cells are digging, building, eating, transporting, communicating and breathing.

As you know by now, the bony struts grow or strengthen according to the needs of the bone of which they are a part. So, again comparing our bones to a city, if a pedestrian bridge were being built, the structure can be constructed with fewer trusses and struts than a bridge that has been built to carry a large locomotive and many boxcars, such as the one shown in photograph 6-d.

Every minute, your bones are responding to their surroundings, reacting in a positive way to good effects or in a negative way to bad influences. For that statement, it follows that it is what a person does every day that determines whether or not their bones will be healthy! If you can, right now, get down on the floor, and do a few push-ups to stimulate your wrist bones!

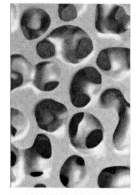

6-e *A close-up view of normal bone*

Normal bone with strong bracing. The truss-like bone is thick and complete.

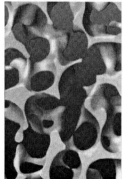

6-f *A close-up view of osteoporotic bone*

The bracing or trusses in this bone affected by osteoporosis are thin, and broken in some places

Kleerekoper M, et al, Calcif Tissue Int. 1985; 37: 594-597

Photographs 6-e and 6-f show animated diagrams of what osteoporotic bone looks like when compared with normal bone. The inner structure, which is trabecular bone, is naturally porous, but the cross braces are solid. Osteoporotic bone, seen in the lower diagram, has slimmer vertical components, as well as some horizontal bracing that has either thinned or separated.

Bone Chemistry A variety of chemicals are found in bone, such as calcium, phosphorus, magnesium, sodium, fluoride, citrates, carbonates, protein, blood, water and — do not be scared off by these names — mucopolysaccharides, which include chondroitin sulphate with glycoproteins and osteopontin (see below).

All the hormones and similar chemicals that control bone strength and growth are found in the rich blood supply. They include vitamin D, estrogen, calcitonin, parathormone, alkaline phosphatase and vitamin C, as well as osteopontin, a hormone that is being studied for its effect upon crystalization.
It is important to note that people who use lead compounds in their hobbies or work are found to have that substance in their bones, along with the normal chemicals.

Supporting Structures of Bone The strength of bone is increased, sometimes considerably, by the soft tissues that coat it, that is, muscle, ligaments, tendons, membranes and skin. It has been found that, compared with the bone of the skull itself, the strength of the skull to resist fractures is increased *fivefold* by the presence of the brain, and the muscles, membranes and skin that cover it.

If we think about it, bone has to be able to resist forces in many ways, compressing down, twisting, stretching, bending, and any combination of these stresses and strains. Obviously, we do need to keep our bone healthy and strong, so that we can stay upright, and thereby help to avoid the misery of fractures.

We know that osteoporosis is important, but who is likely to get it? As we have said, osteoporosis is a disease, and therefore there have to be some causes, and there are certainly many. We do hear a lot about menopause and this disease, and this tends to make people think that it is the only cause for this mostly 'quiet' disorder. Without a doubt, osteoporosis is more common in women than in men. Frequently, we see or hear various medical statements made that declare that about one in four women are affected by this bone-weakening disorder, compared with about one in eight men.

Children can develop osteoporosis as well, which is important for parents to realize. Perhaps we should be asking health practitioners to include a bone assessment as part of the whole family medical examination.

Now, look at the list below to see how you fit in with the risks of having this disease that seemingly ages bone prematurely.

- Are you female gender?

- Do you have a family history of osteoporosis? Yes, your genes, just like workers in a factory or bees in a hive, control the quality of the products made. For example, good quality honey from a beehive is produced by healthy bees that collect good quality pollens and nectar. Your genes control the chemicals that make up bone to be good quality or bad quality. Bad genes, that is, ones that control, in this case, the substances that cause or are associated with osteoporosis can unfortunately be passed on from mother to daughter; in other words, if your mother has or had osteoporosis, then as a daughter you could also develop it.

- Are you close to the age for menopause or beyond (in the case of men, andropause)?

- If you are black-skinned, naturally then you are less likely to suffer osteoporosis than are Asians, Orientals and people with white or light-colored skin.

- As mentioned above, certain chemicals can interfere with the bone 'factory'. Smoking cigarettes, as well as hurting other tissues in the body, is harmful to bone. Excess alcohol is another bad chemical for bone, as are carbonated fizzy pop drinks and certain chemicals designed as medications.

A study performed in Phoenix, Arizona, suggests that excess caffeine does not cause fractures in postmenopausal women, a finding that would suggest that caffeine is not a factor in weakening bone. Many other reports have suggested that caffeine is a cause for osteoporosis, and yet others have shown that caffeine-containing beverages, such as tea, actually strengthen bone. To date, it would seem that caffeine is not a major 'poison' to bone.

The drugs that thin bone should be mentioned, because they do include a well-known cause for osteoporosis — cortisone; however, it is not always dangerous. Cortisone injected into joints is not known to cause osteoporosis, nor is taking a low dose of prednisone (a type of cortisone in common use as a medicine), which means 7.5mg or less for up to three months.

Medication for epilepsy, too much thyroid hormone, and prolonged progesterone (when estrogen is not being used) are other substances that can increase the fragility of bone tissue.

The authors of a small medical study found that excess salt (sodium) can encourage calcium to leave the crystals that make up bone.

- Are you exercising too much? Many young adult women hear that exercise is good for bone, and they also want to look slim. So, what they do is reduce their food intake, and sometimes exercise too much. This combination of low food intake and excess exercise can lead to a medical condition called the *female athletic triad*, which means that these women suffer from three medical states all at the same time: their menstrual cycle ceases, their body weight drops too low, and they develop osteoporosis.

- Is your food quality adequate for good health, including bone health?
  That is, do you have adequate protein, calcium, vitamin D and vitamin C in the food that you eat?
  You do need *enough* protein, but not too much, because this can push out calcium from your bones.

- Are you chronically disabled or, if not disabled, do you tend to sit or lie down too much? In either case, if you do little in the way of weight-bearing exercises, you could be at risk of developing weak bones.

- Do you suffer from other chronic illnesses, such as an overactive thyroid or parathyroid gland, Cushing's disease, or multiple myeloma and other cancers? One rare disease that can weaken bone is primary biliary cirrhosis.

- Are you of advanced age (65+ years)?

- Are you tall and thin, that is, underweight for your height. This, of course, is not your fault, but it puts you at risk for bone fractures. Photograph 6-g is a shadow, but it is hoped that it will remind anyone who is thin to do everything necessary to strengthen their bones and to learn how to avoid fractures.

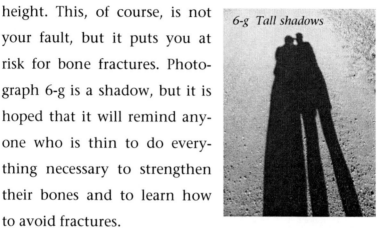

6-g Tall shadows

- Too much sunshine in some individuals can cause certain types of skin cancer. Lack of sunshine can result in low vitamin D levels in the blood, which can be associated with osteoporosis in both children and adults; thus, if you have a risk of skin cancer or have to avoid the sun, you will need all your vitamin D in tablet or liquid form (see comments, in Group F below, on prevention of osteoporosis).

Osteoporosis is not the only disease that can cause bones to break easier than healthy bone. It is beyond the scope of this book to discuss in detail the less common diseases that weaken bone, but osteomalacia and Paget's disease have to be considered as possible causes when a person fractures bones easily.

I hope that you are not part of this story, but if you are do not worry. There are tests available to find out if a person does have fragile bones, as well as other methods of telling when you are at risk or not of suffering from osteoporosis. Your personal medical history and your family medical history are two important starting points in diagnosis. A physical examination is also important, as well as the necessary blood and urine tests. See your physician to discuss the above tests, which would include a blood calcium level, a kidney function test, a bone enzyme test, blood protein tests, and possibly many others. There are also specialized tests, including ultrasound, and a low-dose x-ray technique called DEXA that measures how dense your bones are.

Other testing devices will be used as time passes, which will improve the accuracy of how severe the osteoporosis is and determine whether or not the treatments are working. (Blood and urine tests for this do exist already, and your doctor might have access to them.)

The good news is this. Treatments for osteoporosis are improving, and the list of available treatments is getting longer all the time. Helping to strengthen bone, as you will gather by now, is not just a matter of taking treatments, but it can, of course, be part of it. If by now you believe you are at risk of weaker than average bone, then prevention, as always, has to be attempted. So, how do we do this? We will list the remedies in six groups.

Let us start with the 'easy' first group of preventable causes of 'thin' bone.

Group A: Stop smoking, reduce alcohol and carbonated drinks, and make sure that you are not taking excessive medications, especially of the type listed above.

Group B: If you are not already doing so, perform weight-bearing exercises to improve your physical fitness. You might need to consult a professional person for advice on this matter, but do not make the mistake of overexercising. (There is more information on this topic in the *body fuel* section of Chapter 10 and the *5x5 Mix* sections, Chapters 16 to 20.)

Group C: If you are at the age of menopause (or andropause in the case of men), seek the advice of an expert on the need for estrogen or testosterone replacement, or other hormone replacement therapy.

Group D: Every structure in your body, from your skin and organs to your blood and bones, is made from the food you eat. This means that, if your bones cannot get enough foods that contain the contents of bone, you will have weak bones. So, if your diet contains enough vitamin D, so that you can absorb enough of the calcium that you are going to eat, and enough protein, an important structure of bone, then you are off to a good start. But do not forget, although your food should be low in bad fats (saturated fats), you do need to eat some fats to help your vitamin D to work to its best capacity. The fats that are best for you, for both your heart and your bones, are called the monounsaturates, for example, olive oil and canola oil.

Group E: Related to the advice given above, if you are underweight, seek advice from a physician or other health professional, who can try to determine the cause for your lack of fat or muscle. Just like obesity, being underweight can be a disease or a genetic feature. Eating disorders are not uncommon, and certainly can be helped by one practitioner or another.

Sometimes specialized clinics help, and sometimes they do not. So, if a person has anorexia nervosa or bulimia, there is someone, somewhere who can help that person, whether it be with psychological methods or traditional and not-so-traditional medication therapy. It is my experience in treating bulimic patients who have almost given up with the usual approaches to the management of this serious disorder that leads me to add this additional comment. Patients who tried the psychological- and antidepressant-type therapies without success, rapidly improved by using an older appetite-suppressing medication. Years later, and off their medication, these patients continue to remain free of their desire to binge eat and to force-vomit their food, and although interested in weight control are not abnormally preoccupied with it.

Group F: Get some sunshine, but do not overdo it. Tanning lotions, the ones that contain compounds that protect you from ultraviolet light, can unfortunately prevent the so-called benefits of sunshine, that is, the activation of vitamin D. It is of interest also that, although these lotions prevent the skin from burning, they might not protect against some skin cancers.

There are symptoms of osteoporosis that can be watched for, and the one that most people recognize easily is when they notice that they are getting shorter.

Another important symptom can be mid-back pain, and the presence of this pain suggests that some of the bony fibres in the back bones are actually breaking. Osteoporosis itself does not cause pain. An x-ray taken from a side view of the back can reveal bone breakage of the backbone, but sometimes it is difficult to see. Other tests that can help to diagnose pain in the mid-back are bone scans, CT scans and MRIs.

An important visible sign of osteoporosis, and one that is extremely gradual, is a forward curvature of the upper back; unfortunately, this curvature is not noticed until it is quite severe. Diagram 2-c in Chapter 2 shows how long hair in women can conceal the gradual worsening of this curvature of the spine.

An important thing to remember is this. If a test shows that your bones are growing more dense, it does not necessarily mean that they are less likely to fracture! Only sometimes does it mean that your bones are becoming stronger.

Avoiding or preventing osteoporosis is not as easy for those of you who are white-skinned, who have osteoporosis in the family, who have diseases associated with thin bone, who are elderly and female, and who are not built with a large frame. You cannot simply take away these risky factors. People in this group of fixed risks of osteoporosis first of all have to eliminate all the factors that can possibly be taken away, for example, smoking. Then, combating the risk factors that they have been born with can begin! In the next chapter, I will discuss the methods that we can use to strengthen our bones.

Chapter 7

The Story of Osteoporosis — Part Two — The Way to Stronger Bones

Everything from health magazines, sports newspapers, gyms, physicians, surgeons, governments, television, radio, drugstores, health food stores, and many more kinds of resources claims to have information on treatments for osteoporosis. It is not my intention here to list every possible treatment declared. Those treatments that have been proved, with approved studies, will be described here; any of the treatments not listed here, should be discussed with your health practitioner.

Now, let us look at treatments that not only improve the strength of bone, as shown by various tests, but also reduce fractures (any break in bones).

Before starting prescribed medication, it is important, of course, to make sure that you have enough calcium with vitamin D in your everyday food. If you eat an average amount and quality of food, then you will be taking in about 800mg of calcium daily. Because the average person needs about 1,500mg of calcium daily, you can add the balance of this, in a liquid or solid form, to your diet. A good choice for a solid form of calcium would be calcium citrate tablets.

To help with some common food sources of calcium, refer to photograph 7-a, along with the legend, 7-b, of the food names. The foods are numbered as follows:

1) Oranges	6) Swiss cheese	11) Sardines
2) Chocolate milk	7) Bread	12) Salmon
3) Milk	8) Almonds	13) Chocolate
4) Lentils	9) Molasses	14) Kale
5) Yoghurt	10) Orange juice	15) Chocolate almonds

7-a high calcium foods

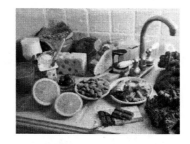

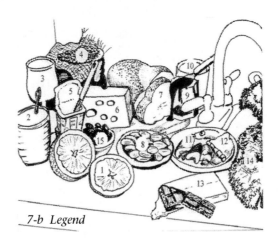

7-b Legend

Now, based upon the latest studies, you also need to have a daily intake of about 800 international units (IU) of vitamin D. As previously mentioned, about half a person's daily vitamin D requirement is activated in the skin by sunshine. This, along with fish liver oils, is the main source of natural vitamin D. Whatever you receive daily in the form of natural vitamin D should be topped up with supplements of this vitamin, so that the total dose adds up to 800 IU daily. For example, if you do have these natural sources of vitamin D, then another 400 IU of this fat soluble vitamin would be enough for an effective daily source.

It is important to point out here that, if you suffer from calcium-type kidney stones, you should include calcium (especially of the citrate type) as part of your treatment. The important part of avoiding this type of kidney stone is keeping to a low *oxalate* diet, and taking enough calcium that it will cling to that oxalate in your intestines, eventually expelling it from the body.

Adequate protein has been mentioned as an important part of your eating plan (fish, poultry, other meats, cheese and eggs are some examples), as well as vitamin C, which helps to make the collagen parts of bone. Try to avoid having *too much* protein for long periods, because this can cause a *loss* of calcium from your bones, as already noted in the above chapter.

Two other important facts to note are the following:

An excess of vitamin A can cause an increase in bone fracture risk.

In men, adequate calcium, with a lack of vitamin D, can increase the risk of prostate cancer.

Treatments, in the form of medications that are prescribed, fall into two groups: those that are *not hormones,* and those that *are hormones.*

The list of non-hormone treatments continues to grow every year. This group of medications can be further divided into smaller groups, each one with its good effects as well as its potential side effects. At least there are choices, so there is usually one that is suitable for you. Some of these treatments are also used to prevent osteoporosis when it is in the osteopenia stage.

To help understand what low bone density means, imagine a piece of bone the size of a golf ball with osteoporosis, and compare it with a golf ball-sized piece of healthy bone. The healthy bone will be the heaviest.

An interesting, but unusual, cause for bone losing calcium, and therefore becoming osteoporotic, is the reduction of gravity.

We all know that astronauts in spaceships that are outside the gravitational pull of planet Earth will develop osteoporosis if they are left in space too long. This has prompted scientists to research osteoporosis from this aspect, and some interesting progress has been made. For example, the vibration of bone procedure, which stimulates bone growth, was discovered by research scientists.

So try to avoid becoming an astronaut if you are a woman over 50 and are not taking estrogen replacement or other treatment for bone thinning!

If you want to impress your friends with long words, learn how to spell this one — *bisphosphonates*. This word is interesting because it was the first family of drugs that were shown to help reduce the progress of osteoporosis and to prevent fractures (bone breakage). There have been various so-called generations of these medicines developed over the years. The early ones were quite weak, but the present-day ones are much stronger. By taking the better quality bisphosphonates, the risk of a fracture will definitely be reduced in people with osteoporosis.

Another important family of medicines are related to drugs that help to prevent the recurrence of breast cancer. These drugs are not hormones, but are related in a way. They actually affect small switches, called receptors, in the body that estrogen hormones attach themselves to. (These medicines have been called 'designer hormones'.) The official name for these important bone-strengthening medications is selective estrogen receptor modulators, which can be shortened to SERMS. They are useful because they help to give the best effects of estrogen while blocking most of the bad effects, especially on the uterus and the breasts. In other words, they help to strengthen bone, can reduce the breast cancer risk, and do not increase the risk of uterine cancer. There is a slight risk, however, of a blood clot disorder with these SERMS, about the same as taking estrogen by mouth. If you have a higher risk than average of a stroke, or of blood clotting in the legs or lungs, you will not be able to take this type of treatment for osteoporosis.

One extremely interesting medication for use in strengthening bone can — believe or not — be sprayed up your nose! We should be thankful to the fish family, especially the salmon, because this is where scientists obtain this medicine. With virtually no side effects, this fine spray is simply squirted up the nose, just once a day. Talk to your physician about this interesting substance that can help both men and women. Pain relief is another useful good effect of this spray, for example, in people in agony from a spinal fracture. In addition, useful for those people who forget to take tablets is an osteoporosis therapy that, at present, is being used to stop calcium loss from bones in patients on certain anti-cancer treatments. This annual injection might be available in the near future as a treatment for almost anyone with osteoporosis.

In the front of the neck, there is a gland called the thyroid. This gland has four neighbors, that is, four tiny glands called the parathyroid glands. These tiny factories release a hormone called parathormone. This substance is now being used for the treatment of osteoporosis, and might well be one of the best treatments available.

Depending on your sex, the next family of treatments is divided into that for women and a separate form for men.

For women, there are many forms of estrogen, and they can, of course, take the treatment listed above. Evidence from various studies suggests that estrogen is not a good *treatment* for osteoporosis.

Along with the various non-hormonal treatments, men can also take testosterone in its various forms — tablets, injections, patches or gels to massage into the skin.

There is more detail on this hormone topic in the chapters on menopause and andropause.

Osteoporosis can occur in animals, and broken bones can obviously occur as well. Interesting animal research (these tests were done in birds) has shown us that vibration with physical methods, such as a vibrating platform, can strengthen bone, so that osteoporosis tends to improve. This vibration system likely benefits all types of bone, including that of human beings. Time and research will give us more information, and will also improve ways for this vibration technology to help to strengthen and heal fractured bone.

A large research group called The Fauna Communications Research Institute (P.O. Box 1126, Hillsborough, N.C, 27278), has reported that they know at least one reason why cats purr. (For the technically minded, the frequency of sound in a domestic cat's purr is about 40Hz.) So far, the findings suggest that the vibration of bone with certain frequencies of sound can actually stimulate the healing of damage to bone. This sound technique is already being tested in human beings, and up to now it seems promising as a treatment for bone healing, and perhaps bone strengthening as well.

So, what does this chapter not deal with? It does not deal with the protection of weak bones or with actual bone injuries. It does not describe the specialized exercises for bone strengthening. In fact, it does not inform you about lots of subjects, such as balance, fall prevention, landing techniques, and other aspects of ways to protect yourself from body damage, and from the many possible injuries that you are exposed to every hour of the day and night.

So, make sure that you read the rest of this book, so that you can understand the following:

The improvement of bone health.

How to strengthen tendons and muscles to further protect bone.

The role of fat in fall injuries.

The prevention of falls.

How to learn landing methods and reflexes to help reduce fracture risks.

The ways to improve balance and posture.

How to improve overall health so that you acquire optimal healing ability.

With this combined knowledge, other positive factors will emerge, including a reduction in the ability of osteoporosis to cause you any harm.

Chapter 8

The Four — *and Three-thirds* — Seasons!

Christmas, springtime, the summer holidays, or fall (autumn) — which is your favorite time of the year? The answer to this question will, of course, vary considerably, depending upon your location on the globe, as well as on your cultural background.

Many countries have four, well-defined seasons of the year: spring, summer, fall (autumn) and winter. Each of these seasons has its own pleasant or desirable features, thus making each one of them attractive to people in a variety of ways. For example, summer is chosen as a favorite time because of its association with warmer weather. Gardeners, campers, older people, the visually handicapped, and many other people, including those who just simply hate cold weather, love the summer for many reasons.

The fall can be, and usually is, a beautiful time of the year. Gorgeous leaf color changes provide a favorite time for photographers, and some individuals, including some animals with thick fur, welcome the cooler temperatures of fall, particularly if the summer has been hot and stormy.

Why would anyone look forward to a winter with snow? Snow means cold weather, and lower than freezing-point temperatures. "Snowbirds" are groups of people who pack their bags at the first hint of cold weather and head for somewhere else, the desert if necessary, anything to get away from those chilly winds that can freeze your flesh in less than a minute. There must be lots of people, such as the snowbirds and those raised in the desert or in tropical lands, whose scalps are raw from the scratching they do while wondering why some of us have an intense love for ice and snow.

It is a fact that some people cannot wait for those freezing temperatures. They long to clamp on their skis or to sharpen their skate blades, so that they can improve on their previous years of sports skills, or just have fun skiing and skating. Climbing frozen waterfalls is actually a passion and a must for some winter enthusiasts.

Whether you enjoy winter or not, spring is almost universally a much welcomed season. The loss of the frosty chill in the air is not missed, and winter is soon forgotten. Those new buds on trees and plants are a sign of warmer days to come, so enthusiasm grows and anticipation mounts for those who love this time of the year and look forward to the many warm-weather activities.

It certainly sounds wonderful. Four fun-filled seasons; it sounds too good to be true … and it is!

Each season, and more, can have its not-so-bright side. Diseases of many types have their favorite time of the year to rear their ugly heads as well. For example, influenza A has a peak time of the year to appear, and these months vary from country to country.

Injuries, as you know by now from what you have already read, are a common event every day of the year. There are times of the year, however, when the different types of trauma have their peak incidence. These peaks also vary from country to country, depending on the weather and the timing of traditional ceremonies and celebrations.

For the sake of simplicity, as well as based on my experience in my practice, the year will be divided into a number of compartments. This chapter assumes the following: winter to be cold and, occasionally at least, below freezing; spring to be the end of winter, and the time for seeds to germinate with the rising soil temperatures; summer to be warm enough for outdoor activities with lightweight clothing; and the fall to be the time when the so-called deciduous trees lose their leaves, and plant growth slows or stops as determined by dropping outside air temperatures.

But apart from these traditional seasons, when looking at the frequency of injuries, one has to consider other times or "seasons" that seem to trigger trauma. These other seasons are the intervals between the traditional seasons, or even within a season itself. They are the three-thirds seasons that I mentioned in the title of this chapter. Before I discuss each in detail, I would like to list them for the sake of clarity. First, there are the One-third (Christmas/New Year) season and the First (Winter) season. These are potentially dangerous times, and they are soon followed by the Two-thirds (February) season. The Second (Spring) season is equally rife with hazards, as is the Third (Summer) season that follows. The Fourth (Fall) season has its share of harmful possibilities, and so does the Three-thirds (Halloween) season that rounds out our potentially perilous year.

The One-third (Christmas/New Year) Season

 If your favorite time happens to be Christmas, then you know that this time, along with New Year's eve, is a peak time for fall-type injuries. Whether it is because of clouding of the mind with the planning involved with this festive time, or from falling off chairs when climbing to decorate trees or locations in your home, or from too much alcohol, or simply because of the weather, this is a peak time to take a tumble or to crash a car.

The First (Winter) Season

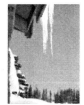

The entire winter itself, of course, is a factor in many injuries. Icy surfaces, long hours of darkness, lower fitness levels, feeling ill from virus-type diseases, blowing snow, visual impairment because of the extensive use of headgear, and a more rigid posture because of the cold are just some reasons why a slip or other type of fall can happen at this time of year.

Unsteady Freddi is shown at a bus stop. She is stiff with cold, and at high risk of a fall because she is standing on ice (see cartoon 8-a).

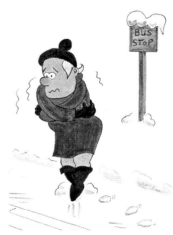

If you remember, my patient at the beginning of this book had a great fear of slipping on the ice and breaking a bone. This fear of falling in itself can increase the chance of a fall.

Winter sports should not be forgotten at this time either.

8-a This shivering woman is too cold to resist a fall

There is a high risk of a variety of injuries in both skiing and skating. Collisions, cuts and falls are the most common trauma seen by medical facilities.

The Two-thirds (February) Season

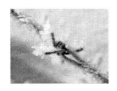 In some countries with snowy winters, February seems to be another in-between time that sees a peak in injuries. Motor vehicle collisions in some regions are reported to be more frequent during this early month of the year as well.

In Canada, early in February is White Cane Week, designated as much by the Canadian Council for the Blind to raise awareness that snow, ice and low temperatures put the blind, as well as other disabled people, at an even greater disadvantage, and that just getting around outside the home is more hazardous because of slippery and cold conditions. At the time of writing, there were no plans for an audio-type presentation of this information, so if you the reader know of people with disabilities please help them to get the best guidance they can. Contact Health Canada or the internet source http://www.canadian-health-network.ca.

For those readers outside Canada, an equivalent department of health will be able to help you.

The Second (Spring) Season

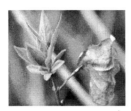

What could sound more innocent than springtime? Spring spills do occur, however, despite the improving daylight and the joy that is traditionally associated with this time.

Loose gravel on travel surfaces, winter debris, and bringing out the bicycle for a quick ride around the block to get fit can combine to result in a spring tumble. Be extra careful with climbing that ladder to fix a loose roof tile or shingle and beware of the surprise of spring snowstorms. Just when you think that winter is safely behind you, it can suddenly reappear as a springtime blizzard!

Photograph 8-b shows a rest between storms, snow having blasted the fields with a springtime blizzard in the western prairies of Canada.

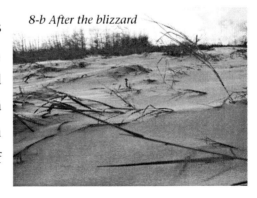

8-b After the blizzard

The Third (Summer) Season

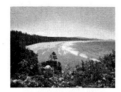

Summertime is a time for just about every type of injury described in the family "injury tree" that appeared earlier in the book to occur. A list should suffice as a reminder that, although it is a favorite time of year, it is not a good idea to switch off your defense systems because you have been encouraged by the ideas of injury prevention outlined between the covers of this book.

Injuries connected with summer include the following:

Burns: The use of outdoor fires is more common, barbecues included, and sunburn and heatstroke in higher outdoor temperatures are a risk.

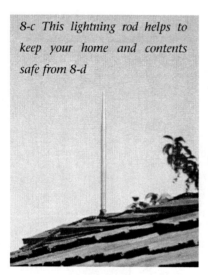

8-c *This lightning rod helps to keep your home and contents safe from 8-d*

Lightning: Try to understand lightning strikes, and how to avoid being struck by one of these potentially lethal natural occurrences. Photograph 8-c shows a lightning rod on the roof of a house. This device helps convert a house from 98% to 100% safe.

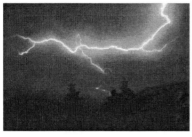

8-d This lightning bolt can really brighten the sky

Photograph 8-d was taken from the safety of the house with the lightning rod, and of course shows an electrical storm with the dreaded lightning bolt.

Farm accidents: These are more likely to happen in the summer, with more machinery-related activities occurring with the growing of crops and the breeding of livestock.

Watercraft mishaps: Boating injuries, along with drownings, are all seen more frequently because of the call of the cooling activities on lakes or in swimming pools.

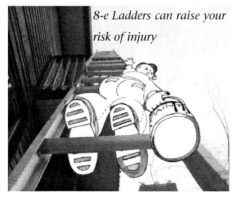

8-e Ladders can raise your risk of injury

Ladders: Falling off ladders can, of course, lead to serious injuries. When climbing ladders, every precaution possible has to be considered to minimize the risk of falling off. Apart from the human precautions (alertness, correct footwear and clothing, etc), use a good quality ladder, ensure that the ladder is stabilized with ropes, and lean it at a safe angle to the surface that it is resting against. Photograph/cartoon 8-e depicts someone climbing a ladder while carrying a can of paint. Anyone who uses paint needs a brush, a cloth, and perhaps reading glasses to see the instructions on the can. All this adds up to an injury risk; imagine a strong wind blowing while at the top of the ladder!

For that matter, building a structure and all types of repair work have their own specific risks of injuries (tools, projectiles, electricity, volatile fluids, etc).

Holiday travel: Both parents and children travel more in the summer, and because of this are exposed to a bigger variety of dangers. Motor vehicle accidents, cuts, falls, plant poisonings, burns, animal attacks, and other trauma listed on the family "injury tree" will be seen more commonly on family trips.

Please know where your children are at every moment, because in a second they can fall off a ledge or into any danger, even — as we hear far too often — get carried off by a stranger. Does every child have a guardian close by in the children's festival (see photograph 8-f)?

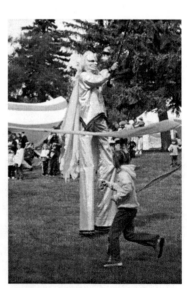

8-f It is easy to get lost at busy events

Outdoor sports: Activities such as tennis, football and baseball, or just jogging, and even golf, help to fill medical emergency departments and doctors' clinics with injuries peculiar to those sports.

Dogs: Apart from just falling off a bicycle, people can be easily pushed over by an off-leash dog. A stray or an aggressive neighborhood dog can charge your bicycle, causing you to fall off without even touching you. The simple fear of being bitten or dragged off the bicycle can cause you to lose control and crash, often causing a nasty-fall-from-a-height injury.

The Three-thirds (Halloween) Season

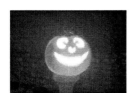

North American communities, along with some European countries, celebrate Halloween on October 31. Those people who construct elaborate Halloween displays to entertain both children and adults can fall off ladders or cut themselves preparing for the celebration. Clothes catching fire and intentional poisonings are not particularly rare at this time of the year either.

The Fourth (Fall) Season

Going from summer to fall means lots of changes for some people who need an abundance of natural light in their lives. At the approach of the end of summer, and especially for those for whom it is a favorite time, the reduction of light can trigger mood disorders. Seasonal affective disorder (SAD), a condition where depression is a significant feature, can include the added complication of fall fractures. Full-spectrum lighting is one of the possible remedies for this mood disorder, and this in turn could reduce the chances of falling over. (This, to my knowledge, has not yet been studied.)

Slipping and sliding are commonly caused by ground conditions that favor this type of fall. Dead, slippery leaves on the ground, new ice from frosts or early cold snaps, and the reduced visibility already mentioned are the conditions people have to adapt to following a season of warm bright conditions.

Both children and adults are at risk of fall and collision injuries because of the darkness, and children are particularly vulnerable because of their costume headgear. Masks and cold-preventing clothing can be at fault for obstructing and reducing surround vision. There are articles that one can read on surround vision and dark adaptation.

In addition, the Block Parents organization has produced a pamphlet on Halloween safety. It is readily available on their Internet site.

Let us look at another example of a celebratory but dangerous time. In the United Kingdom, Guy Fawkes Night, as it is called, is a scary time for many parents and grandparents, and a busy time for hospitals and fire departments.

The fireworks used by many families at this time of the year, November 5, present a fire and explosion risk, and have the ability to cause severe burns, along with the loss of limbs and eyes. The scale of damage can run from singed hair and scorched clothing to houses set on fire!

Additional Noteworthy Tips for Movement on Foot

Walking in the dark at night, as everyone knows, can be risky. Reduced light not only affects the vision but can also confuse or disorient a person to their surroundings; moreover, nighttime has its own peculiar type of life, which in turn can create further dangers. In both city and rural areas, drunk drivers are always around, along with the villains who are responsible for the robbery and intentional assault-type injuries.

Walking on hills and slopes, near deep water, on ice, on loose rocks, and through heavy vegetation all have their obvious dangers.

Movement around the home in the dark also presents similar risks to the outdoors. Tripping over objects and falling down the stairs are some of the more obvious risks.

The risks of falls at night can all be reduced with care and attention. First, follow all the general rules of injury prevention: correct clothing is necessary for the dark, all your special senses should be on high alert, and you should allow your eyes to adapt to the dark before proceeding. When moving from a well-lighted area to a dark location, your eyes need time for the pupils to open up and for the retinae of the eyes to switch on the nerve endings that are designed to work more effectively in the dark. This process starts to work immediately, but can take up to half an hour or so to reach maximum efficiency. Most people cannot wait more than half an hour to start walking out into the night after leaving a lighted area. It is strongly advised, however, to stand still for at least two minutes before walking into the complete darkness.

If there are bright lights around you that are not illuminating your way or the general area in which you are walking, try to avoid staring at them, because these sources of useless light only constrict your pupils, thereby reducing the useful light that is helping you to see your surroundings. Another way of putting this is that useless light prevents you from adapting to the dark. Common examples of useless light could be distant streetlights, car headlights or lights in distant homes.

On cold and windy days, the eyes tend to produce excess tears to prevent them from drying out too much. Tearing of the eyes does settle once they have adapted to adverse cold and windy conditions, but while adapting there is a short time when your vision will be reduced by those tears, thus increasing the risk of a collision, fall or other accident.

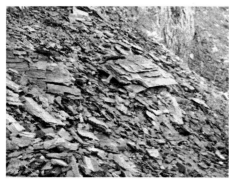

8-g One of the most slippery surfaces, especially when wet

Travel in forests and mountains has many risks as well. The most slippery surface encountered anywhere in summer or winter in the mountains is scree. These plates of rock can slide over each other extremely easily, and they are almost impossible to walk on without sliding. Usually, there is an incline as part of the terrain, making any fall from this location even more likely and even more serious. Do not try to walk on scree unless it is absolutely

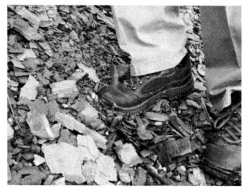

unavoidable. Photographs 8-g and 8-h show that risky scree surface, as slippery as ice!

8-h Scree can drop you quicker than ice

In situations where you have to walk down a steep slope, on a hill for example, try to descend by moving in a zigzag pattern. Keep your knees flexed (bent), your arms supple and hanging low, as if ready to fall, and use your eyes to peak efficiency. When descending, keep your spine upright, but when walking uphill relax it in a forward position. Using a zigzag pattern while walking downhill ensures that the incline you follow is minimal, and that if you do fall it will be to your side, except when changing direction.

Loose rock, tree roots and slippery clay are just a few of the many other surface risks that can cause a fall. These can be avoided by simply keeping your eyes peeled, and by using the skills that you can acquire in the *5x5 Mix* exercises and other principles of fall prevention.

Beware of prolonged activity fatigue! On long hikes, for example, if you are unfit, or as you tire from climbing slopes,

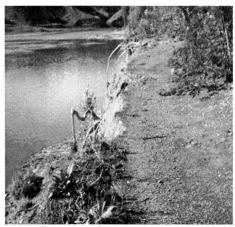 especially at high altitudes, your legs will weaken, your ability or tendency to lift your feet will be reduced, and a trip over rocks or something similar will be more likely.

8-i This river edge is an extremely dangerous place, especially after a heavy rainfall

Avalanches, flash-floods, lightning from sudden storms, fog, snowstorms, heavy rain, hunters and certain types of wildlife are some other causes of trauma or death.

Nothing in the discussion above, however, should discourage anyone from walking activities or sports. It is just that being aware of the locations of and the causes for the many types of fall and other types of injuries, and knowing how to prevent or arm yourself against them, can have a major impact on how you can avoid the suffering, the pain, and the disability or worse that can result from any type of trauma.

Remember, even though we have been discussing the perils of the outdoors, most injuries still do occur *indoors*. If you are older and confined to the indoors, falling over in your own house is a common cause of broken bones, a condition that can kill you! Falls in the kitchen and down the stairs are some of the most common ways and places to hurt yourself. Take all the precautions that have been recommended in this book, and those suggested by your own medical doctor. For example, get help with keeping the floor clear of objects that can cause you to trip, use aids in the bathroom to prevent slips, wear shoes that fit and grip well, use your eyes and ears to the best of their ability (and get medical help with those special senses if it is necessary), do not wear loose clothing that can catch on objects, avoid alcohol and medicine that makes you light-headed, and have regular medical checkups to help with any symptoms that can weaken you. For those people who use reading or bifocal glasses, be careful walking, especially when going down the stairs.

If you are weak, certain exercises can help you to become stronger, even if you are more than 90 years of age!

Combine all the *awareness ideas with skills in landing* and you will have close to *a perfect injury avoidance formula!*

Chapter 9

The Six-minute Self-breast Examination — The Correct Way!

For convenience, I will be using the term self-breast exam (SBE), to refer to a breast examination done by you. The correct term is breast self-examination, or BSE; however, this initialism has unfortunately achieved a certain notoriety recently because it can also mean bovine spongioform encephalopathy (mad cow disease)!

Know your four armpit triangles, as well as the usual difference between a serious breast growth and a non-life-threatening lump.

The discussion below describes how *all* breast lumps are important until a biopsy has shown the true nature of the growth that was found. This information is here to help cut the chances of you dying young, unnecessarily and prematurely.

If you do not know how to do a *correct* self-breast examination, then please read and understand this information and follow the directions carefully. I hope that you will make this procedure a *monthly habit!*

Just as injury prevention is taught to reduce unnecessary death or suffering, the information shown here is designed to find a breast cancer as early as possible, thereby making a cure more likely. Thus, the possibility of a premature death or unpleasant treatments could be reduced or even avoided altogether simply by using a hand! If that hand, your own or that of someone else (preferably your doctor, your husband, or an extremely close friend!), knows the skills taught here it is quite possible to find a breast lump as small as a *grain of rice!*

Details of the breast cancer disease are not presented here. This is so I can concentrate on emphasizing this most important preventive technique. This method comprises *five* stages or steps, and you should take at least six minutes to complete this self-breast examination technique successfully.

First, remove your upper clothing, and please note that these directions assume that the reader has reasonably good vision and the use of both hands and upper limbs. Obviously, if this not the case, then another person will have to help you with this exam.

The five steps of a complete self-breast examination are as follows:

Part One — Look

Standing, if possible, look in a mirror so that you can see your breasts clearly, and then follow these easy steps. From the standing position, raise your arms straight up until they are pointing toward the sky — your breasts will rise a little.

Lower your arms so that they are pointing out from your body, aimed slightly downward to the floor — at this point, the breasts will be pushed together.

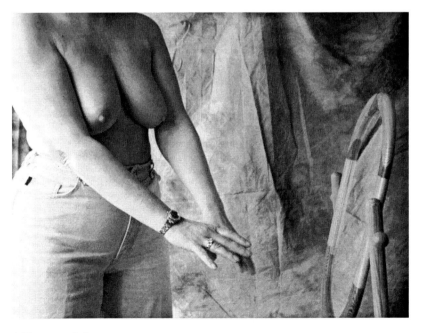

Photograph 9-a

Photograph 9-a shows the position of your breasts and arms described so far.

Push each arm up and back as far as possible, as if you are stretching the chest muscles; the breasts are pulled outward at this point, as seen in photograph 9-b.

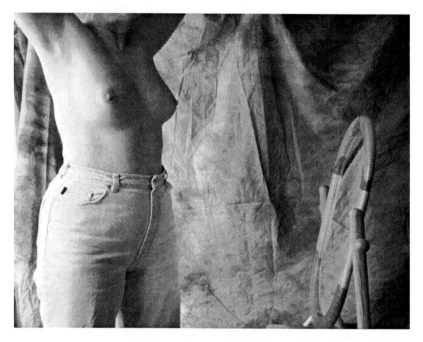

Photograph 9-b

The final step of checking the breast appearance is to simply bend forward so that your arms hang freely downward toward the floor; both breasts should also hang, nipples pointing down.

Photograph 9-c shows this hanging breast view.

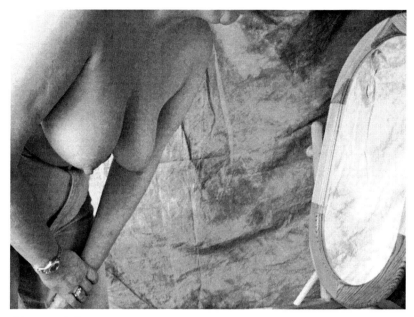

Photograph 9-c

Throughout these five recommended steps, watch for any of the following possible findings:

- Skin rashes; black moles; red, scaly patches; and oozing, irritated skin in the nipple area or in the breast regions. Actually, this is a good time to inspect the entire body for these signs of skin cancer.

- A change in nipple appearance, such as the nipples pointing in a different direction to what you are used to seeing, a sinking-in (retracted) nipple, or a discharge of any type.

- Skin creases (especially when closing your out-stretched arms, that is, when bringing your hands together); this skin sign looks as if the breast is folding in, creating this groove in the surface skin.

- Dimpling of the breast skin can look like the surface of an orange, and can best be seen when the breast is being stretched, that is, when you reach out with your arms. Technically, this orange peel appearance is called by the French term for "orange skin," *peau d'orange,* and it is, of course, abnormal and can be caused by a cancerous growth.

- A persistent boil or abscess in the breast needs to be investigated to check for a cancerous cause.

Anything different in your breast appearance that is not mentioned above, as well as any of the changes above, should be checked by a doctor.

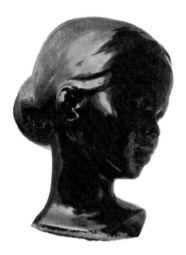

Part Two — Touch

Part Two of this self-breast examination is best done lying down face up on your back in as relaxed and as comfortable a position as possible. In the above position, the body is more relaxed, and the breast tissue is more evenly spread out over the chest wall.

Using the fingertips, that is, the pads of two or three fingers, make small circular movements, with enough pressure to indent the breast flesh, so that the glandular structures are felt; make sure, of course, that the tips of your nails do not indent the skin.

Photograph 9-d shows a front view of the fingers used in the Part Two examination; the little finger does not usually make contact with breast structures.

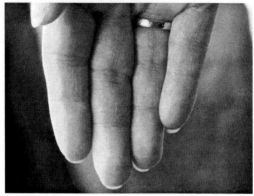

Photograph 9-d

Press gently over the notch at the top of the breastbone, and then run your fingers along the underside of the collarbone until the shoulder is reached.

This start position is shown in photograph 9-e.

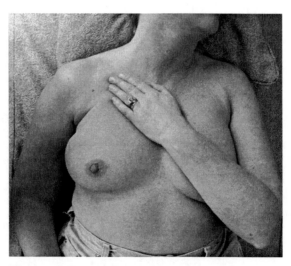

Photograph 9-e

Now run your fingers down the outer side of the breast, following the curve of the lower edge of the breast inward until your fingertips reach the lower end of the breastbone — your fingertips should be between the lower edge of each breast.

Now push the fingertips upward along the middle of the chest, back to the notch at the top of the breastbone where you started. At this point, you have simply run your fingers around the outside edge of one breast, moving them in the continuous small circles described above.

The next step is to continue to gently run your fingertips on in the same direction, in spiraling decreasing circular movements, until the nipple is reached.

Make sure that you overlap the area of breast tissue felt as you spiral inward, so that every square inch of the breast is covered by this self-check method.

Photograph 9-f shows that part where the fingertips have reached the lower outside edge of the right breast and are approaching the midline of the chest.

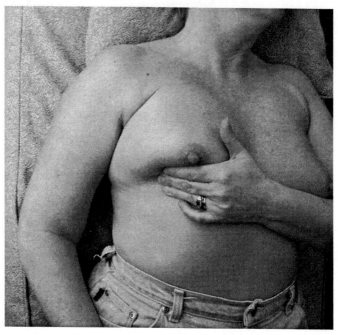

Photograph 9-f

For extremely large breasts, this process should be repeated three times: the first circuit with gentle pressure, the second with more pressure, and the third with enough pressure to reach the deeper breast tissues.

Repeat this method on the other breast using the opposite hand (right hand for the left breast; left hand for the right).

With this part of the exam, you are looking for any lump that is not part of the normal breast glandular tissue.

There are at least three regions of the breast where cancers can hide.

1) Just below the collarbone

2) Behind the nipple

3) In the armpit

So, check these areas of the breast with a strong determination to seek out hidden growths.

Normal breast tissue is made up of clumps of glandular tissue called lobes, each one with a duct. There are 10 to 20 of these lobes in each breast, and each one is further divided into many smaller units called lobules. These lobes and ducts are covered in fat, and as normal breast parts they can feel lumpy all the time or only at certain times of the month. Most of the time, these lumpy areas can be held with the fingers and be moved around quite freely, because they are not attached to the ribs or muscles of the chest wall.

As you repeat this examination many times, try to memorize the normal pattern of your breast. Some regions might feel thicker or denser than other areas, and some might be more tender; again, this can depend on the time of the month that you examine yourself. If you are ever doubtful about this examination method, or if you are unsure about what you are feeling, have your personal doctor repeat the procedure for you.

Part Three — Feel

As above, Part Three of the six-minute examination should be carried out in a relaxed position while lying on your back. For this important part, you use either the entire surface of the front of the hand or just the surface of the four fingers, depending on the amount of fat in the breast.

This palm pressure method is not a replacement for Part Two of the examination, it is in addition to it. The palm of the hand detects different textures than the fingertips, often picking out the more serious types of lumps from the more normal lumpy lobular tissue. With the palm, you should combine a sweeping motion, with a circular-type action as the hand presses into the breast tissues.

Photograph 9-g is a reminder to use as large an area as possible of the hand to examine and compare bigger breast sections.

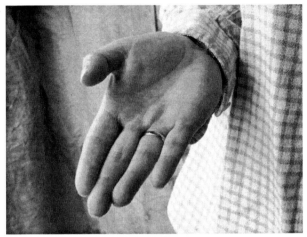

Photograph 9-g

By covering a larger area of the breast surface, the fingers, and palm if necessary, are automatically comparing separate bunches of lobules, and are able to pick up lumps that are not as mobile as other more normal breast glands.

Just imagine the breast being divided up into four sections, with the nipple being the center. These sections can be called the top outer, the top inner, the bottom inner and the bottom outer.

Place the pads of your fingers, with the upper palm of your hand in contact with the breast, over one of these quarter sections, and press into the skin until you can feel the glandular structures. With small, circular sweeping move-

ments, feel the ducts and glands, moving your hand continually, until the whole quarter section of the breast has
been covered, and then, of course, move on to the other
three sections of the breast, repeating the same moves.

Photograph 9-h shows the hand placement to examine approximately one quarter section of the breast.

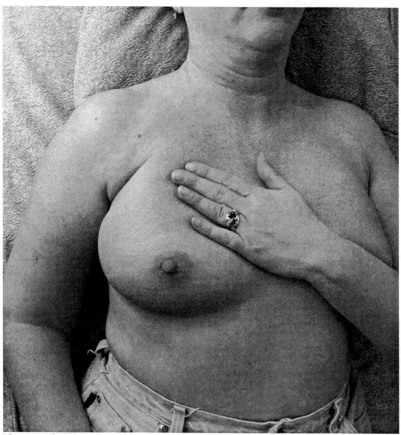

Photograph 9-h

For the other breast, the above procedure is the same. As in Part Two, use your left hand for the right breast and your right hand for the left. If you have had an upper limb removal or cannot use a hand for some reason, have either your doctor check you monthly or a friend or partner learn this breast examination method so that they can help you.

This finger and palm method is used to seek out any size lump that is *not* normal breast tissue. Normal structures move fairly freely, and so make sure, as you gently grip the breast structures, that they move with the circular and sweeping palm and finger actions. Once you are used to the normal structures moving across the chest wall smoothly, you will easily detect any lump that is fixed or non-moveable. (See the list of typical breast cancer features at the end of this chapter.)

If the breast is small and naturally quite lumpy, the lobes will be extremely difficult, if not impossible, to move around, in which case only a medical expert should be in charge of the breast surveillance.

Some cancers can be more of a rubbery texture and seem to move a little when pushed, tending to rock from side to side.

Always get each breast lump checked by a doctor, because, although many cancers are typical, there are many varieties that can fool anyone.

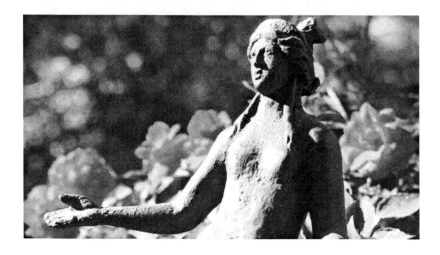

Part Four — The Nipple

Whether you have one, two, four or even six nipples, it is worth devoting an entire part of the self-breast examination to the extremely important nipple.

Photograph 9-i shows, of course, a nipple, but it is a reminder to look at the nipple, first watching for changes in nipple position, and then for the presence of rashes in this region. Cancer of the nipple skin can show itself as a rash.

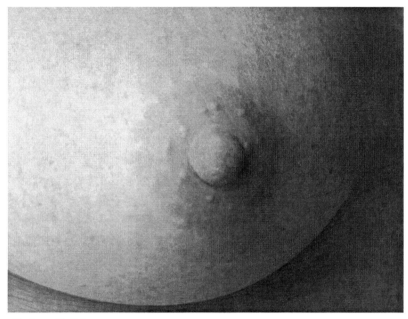

Photograph 9-i

In Part One of this breast examination, the nipple was in-
spected; in this part, it has to be squeezed. Simply take the
whole nipple between the thumb and index finger, gripping well behind it into the breast ducts. Work the fingers
around the nipple, until every piece of skin, and the underlying ducts and glands, have been squeezed.

Photographs 9-j and 9-k both demonstrate a way to compress behind the nipple.

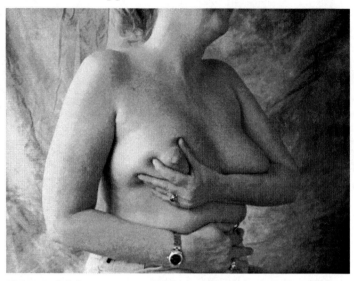

Photograph 9-j

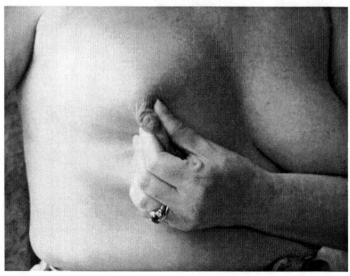

Photograph 9-k

Cancers in the nipple do occur, and they are often hard when felt. Frequently, they can cause the nipple to be drawn inward (indented or retracted). Approximately one in six or seven breast cancers can hide behind the nipple.

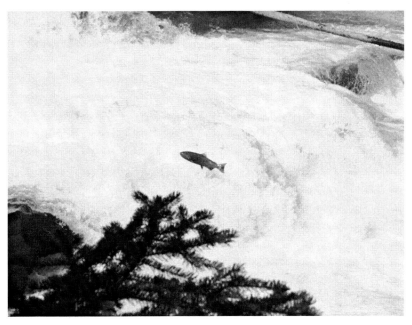

Conditions in nature are always changing, so, if you keep watching you might find unexpected events such as in this photograph, a salmon leaping out of a stream. On one day the breast might be lump-free, a month later a growth could appear!

Part Five — The Armpit

The hollow space between your upper arm and your chest wall and ribs is an important area to examine. Before doing this check, you should understand the normal parts of the armpit (its technical name is the axilla, and it is shown in photograph 9-1).

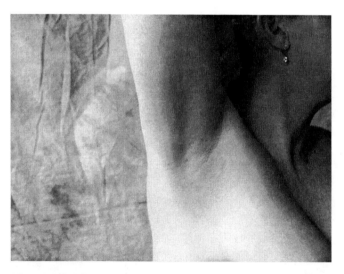

Photograph 9-1

There are five parts or areas to check in the armpit, and all are arranged somewhat like the shape of a pyramid, having four triangular walls and a peak. The following description will help you to understand how the four sides of the armpit are found or arranged, and how you can inspect these four walls and the peak of the armpit pyramid.

Sitting is a good starting position, with one hand resting on your waist.

Wall 1: The front wall of the armpit includes a part of the breast called the tail, which lies over the pectoral or wing muscle of the chest. Using your other hand, first grip the breast tail between your thumb and other fingers. This axillary tail is that part of the breast that spreads up and out from the mammary glandular tissue to the armpit. If you imagine the breast as a teardrop shape, then the pointy part is the one that you are examining. As you grip this area, the edge of the pectoral muscle is being checked at the same time. Run your fingers along the upper to lower armpit edge (see photograph 9-m and 9-q).

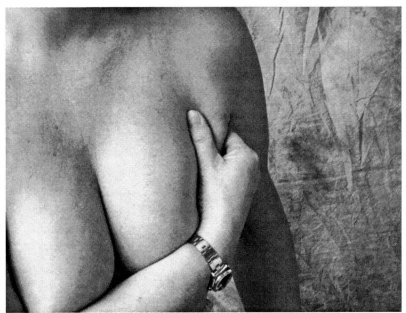

Photograph 9-m

Wall 2: The back wall of the armpit can be felt next. This wall is made up of the muscles that stretch from the ribs up to the back of the arm, and the main muscle is called the latissimus dorsi. Here, with your thumb resting against the front part of the back wall, grip along the shoulder blade region with your other fingers. Again, run your thumb up and down this armpit edge (see photograph 9-n and 9-q).

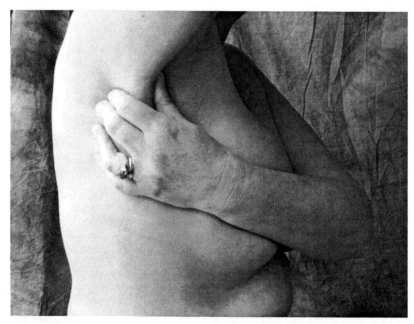

Photograph 9-n

Wall 3: The inside wall of the armpit is made up of the chest wall, that is, the rib surface. To check it, simply press the fingertips down from the top of the armpit, and then stroke them over the rib side, that is, the inner surface between the back and front walls (see photograph 9-o and 9-q).

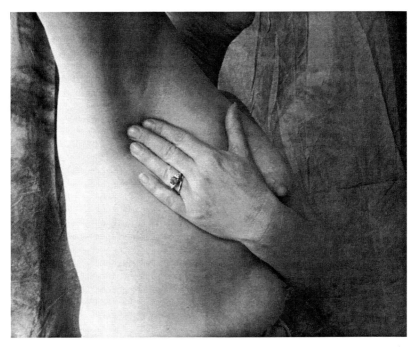

Photograph 9-o

Wall 4: The outer wall of the armpit is found on the *inside* of the upper arm. Using your fingertips, run along the top of the armpit, and then down the inner edge of the upper arm. The distance that needs to be examined down this inner side of the arm is about the width of your hand. Your thumb can rest just below the shoulder or point upward (Photograph 9-p shows this fourth part of the armpit checkup. See also 9-q.)

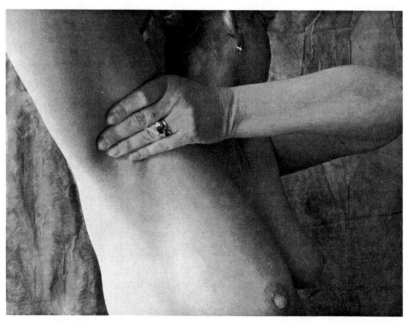

Photograph 9-p

The fifth part of this armpit examination is really a double check. It consists of probing the inside peak, the final region to be felt. Using your fingertips, stroke the highest point in the armpit — this is where the four walls meet at the peak of this pyramid-shaped space. (Photograph 9-q shows the peak of the pyramid-shaped armpit.)

Make sure that both armpits are included, and as in the rest of this breast checkup any type of lump is being looked for anywhere. Various types of lumps can be found in the armpit, and it is just as important to self-examine as the breast itself.

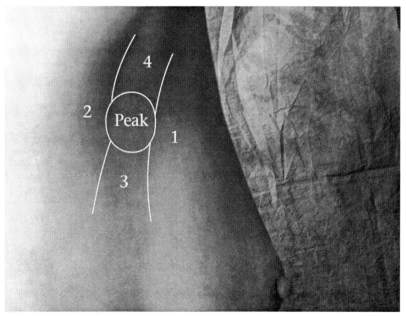

Photograph 9-q Armpit walls 1,2,3,4, and peak

Because the armpits get daily attention, with the use of deodorants and the regular stripping of hair, a monthly lump checkup should not be too much to expect. Armpits can be homes for normal clumps of breast tissue, as well as for different types of cancers (many of which are curable though if caught early), along with frequently found lymph nodes. As before, anything found — lumps, rashes, unusual moles — in this important area of the body needs to be checked by your doctor.

The final part of this chapter will attempt to compare a simple benign, that is, non-cancerous lump with a more serious cancerous lump.

By way of clarification, the term fixed lump should be explained in more detail.

When a breast thickening is found, the mass can be totally free to move around with your fingers, adhering neither to the skin above nor the chest surface below. For example, if the lump is part of the nipple, it will be impossible to move this abnormal breast mass without the nipple moving with it. In the same way, a growth might be clinging to the surface of the chest wall (muscle and ribs with a membranous covering). When you try to push one of these fixed lumps with your fingers, it will either rock back and forth, or not move at all.

A summary in list form comparing breast lump types is shown on the next page.

It is important to note that the only way to be sure whether a lump in the breast or in the armpit, or for that matter in any part of the body, is cancerous or not is by having what is called a *biopsy*. A biopsy is a procedure where a piece of a lump — if possible the whole lump — is taken, either by a surgical method or by the use of a special needle. Parts of the lump taken from the breast or armpit are then examined under a microscope for cancer cells.

Be aware that a mammogram cannot guarantee that a lump is benign and therefore non-cancerous. Anyone who has a new or even slightly suspicious breast lump should have a breast lump biopsy. If you are worried about any breast lump, you should *insist on having a biopsy, even if your mammogram indicates that there is no cancer or lump of any type to be seen anywhere!*

Breast Lump Types

Possible Serious Types

- Fixed/does not move
- Not tender
- Usually feels rough
- Appears gradually
- Slowly gets bigger
- Skin or nipple can be distorted
- Oval, but hard to the touch.

Usually Safe

- Moves easily but can rock
- Tender
- Smooth to the touch when felt
- Oval, but soft or firm
- Appears suddenly
- Varies in size
- Skin above the lump is smooth

A Note To Keep in Mind

If you have regular mammograms, ask the technician to inform you how high the dose of radiation that you are being exposed to is.

A chest x-ray is considered safe. A mammogram, however, can expose you to nearly 1000 times more x-rays than a chest x-ray. Imagine the radiation dose that you would receive if the technician were to repeat your mammogram — once, or even twice. More alarmingly, this actually happens in some clinics! (See Professor Epstein's information below.)

Most cancer clinics suggest that mammograms, as a *screening* test, be carried out every two years between the ages of 50 to 69 years.

To help diagnose an abnormal breast condition, a lump or a breast skin distortion, a mammogram and ultrasound are often used to try to predict whether the need for a biopsy is urgent or not. As mentioned above though, all lumps should be tested under the microscope to determine what type of cells are present in them.

To summarize a mammogram finding:

If a mammogram suggests cancer, get a biopsy.

If a mammogram suggests that a lump in the breast is not cancer, still get a biopsy.

More Information on Mammograms

Please be reminded that a large study suggested that *screening* mammograms do not reduce the death rates from breast cancer. The National Breast Screening Study-2 (there was, as suggested, a previous study of the same name), compared almost 40,000 women with breast cancer screening methods. These women, in their fifties, were divided into two groups. Half the group were regularly examined for breast cancer (by the person themselves and by an expert). The other half were examined and had a mammogram. At the end of this five-year study, the deaths from breast cancer were compared in these two groups. It was shown, as in the first study, that the death rates were about the same. In fact, when recorded in 1996, 107 women died who had mammograms with an examination, whereas 105 lost their lives to breast cancer where the x-rays were not used for the screening process. For more details, see the University of Toronto website on this topic.

Certainly, mammograms have found breast cancers and have saved lives, but they also miss cancers, giving some women a false sense of safety and therefore contributing to their deaths. As before, if a lump is found in the breast, it should be biopsied, or, if you would prefer a non-invasive test before a surgical procedure is considered, an MRI is more accurate than a mammogram.

Professor Samuel Epstein of the Department of Environmental Medicine and School of Public Health, University of Illinois, Chicago, who is also the chairman of the Cancer Prevention Coalition, states that mammograms should be avoided if at all possible. He maintains that they are potentially dangerous, and agrees with the University of Toronto study that mammograms do not save lives overall.

As a physician who has observed women for breast cancer for close to thirty years, I have seen my share of false-positive and false-negative mammograms, all of which have had significant psychological effects on the patients and their families. Along with other medical practitioners, I would welcome a better screening method for breast cancer than mammograms, but in the meantime a woman examining her own breasts is an efficient and safe way to find early breast cancer!

Chapter 10

Fish, Flavonoids and Feeding Facts on the Body's Finest Fuels

Dedicated to human beings — both female and male

Too many people suffer from the top five preventable causes that can end your life early. The diseases that cause premature death can be — have to be — reduced to a lower level than they are at present.

To cut the misery of the aftereffects of heart attacks and strokes, cancers and injuries, as well as to prevent premature death, you, the reader, will have to make changes in your life regularly and learn and practise new ideas.

Read this information on human fuel, that is, food and drink, and combine it with the injury avoidance guide *to achieve a high resistance* to the top three killers. Yes, you do have to practise what I preach though to gain this advantage.

It is hoped that any confusion in nutrition terms that you have encountered in your past or present reading will be settled with the information provided below.
The art of nutrition is eating the type of food that allows your healthy body parts to stay healthy and to resist all

disease, and at the same time help you to feel energetic and well.

Fashions and fads do exist in the world of nutrition, and these are created by health food stores, by the media, and even by some doctors who practise more alternative medicine than regular so-called evidence-based medicine (this is the 'in' term currently used by 'us' doctors). Most products promoted by complimentary health companies are not harmful, in fact, some are actually good for you!

The principle of good nutrition is really this:
It is the type of food that has been *proved to prolong life* that really shows itself as the best diet to be a part of your regular eating plan.

If you need information on the substances that you hear about, such as antioxidants, homocysteine, flavonoids, omega-3 or omega-6, and many other technical names that you are told you need, see a person truly qualified to give the correct information. Dietitians, medical doctors, and even students of science can fill you in with better information than a salesperson in a store or health shop. This chapter does explain many useful dietary words.

The Diseases that Are Likely To Kill You

What are the *diseases* that are likely to kill you? (Keep in mind that, if a disease does not get you, old age eventually will!)

These are the top three killer diseases:

Heart attacks continue to kill more women than any other malady, although the number of deaths in some parts of the world is reducing. The cessation of smoking, better eating, more exercise and improving medical treatments are the major reasons for this drop.

Colon and lung cancers take second place as the next biggest killer in most parts of the world.

Injuries, as you know by now from your reading of this book, are our third biggest enemy as a reason for suffering and dying. For those below forty-four years of age, injuries are the top-of-the-list killer!

Because we are now discussing the primary reasons for dying, let us also look at which women live the longest and why they are able to do so.

It is well-known among doctors that the Mediterranean diet is one of the healthiest ways to eat, and a recent scientific report (from Sweden) suggests that it even seems to reduce the symptoms of rheumatoid arthritis. According to the United Nations, although women in countries that border or are located in the Mediterranean Sea, such as Crete, have a good life expectancy when compared with that of women from, say, Scotland, worldwide it is Japanese women who live the longest!

Is rice wine (sake) a better life preserver than red wine?

Perhaps the line of latitude is a factor.

Is Japanese food superior to Mediterranean food?

Does genetics, or even body size, have a part to play in longer life expectancy for Japanese women?

Before looking at why Japanese women live longer, I shall list some foods that are known to work well in helping to prevent the most common causes for the diseases most likely to kill.

Heart attacks are caused by the blockage of a blood vessel that supplies blood to the heart muscle. The blockage is made up of fats, such as bad cholesterol, and blood particles (from the clotting process), along with other substances, including virus-like agents. This cutoff of the blood supply to the heart can cause heart muscle damage, as well as deadly irregular rhythms of the heartbeat.

A good balance of preventive actions, despite genetics, can go a long way to stop heart attacks: moderate exercise, relaxation, the correct food intake, and controlling as perfectly as possible those other diseases that raise your risk of a heart attack, such as high blood pressure and diabetes. Stopping smoking is essential. This list can, of course, be extended.

A good heart diet will lower your bad cholesterol, protect you from that same bad cholesterol, preserve heart muscle, and prevent an irregular heartbeat. As this type of eating is followed, one should also take care with foods that are bad for the blood pressure, blood sugar, gout, kidney stones and other diseases.

Foods that Are a Good Choice for the Heart

Fatty Fish: Sardines, mackerel, Arctic char, salmon, herring, bluefish and others can be chosen for any meal of the day. Swordfish could be listed as well, but because of the overfishing of this species please choose from the other more plentiful fish species when buying your groceries.

A variety of fish each week is a good way to eat this excellent choice of protein. By eating different species of fish, moreover, you will avoid the same toxins that some fish have been found to contain, because not all fish contain high levels of mercury. Farmed salmon should be avoided because of their association with a variety of noxious agents. So, choose wild salmon.

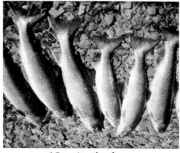

The fish listed here are a high source of the famous omega-3 fatty acids (see photograph 10-a, the fresh catch of the day — Arctic char, courtesy Laurie Serink).

10-a Arctic char

Omega-3 polyunsaturated fatty acids, which are essential in the body as either a lipid or a fat, not only protect your heart from bad cholesterol but also help to prevent fatal irregular heartbeats. The prevention of blood clots and the lowering of the bad blood fats (triglycerides) are other desirable effects (see the Glossary for more information on fats).

Bottled omega-3 oils are available in a capsule form. These preparations have been found to be effective in reducing heart attacks. It is not yet known if they are as effective as the whole fish, but if pure, that is, if they contain no fish proteins, they could be useful in those people with fish allergies. Those people with fish allergies, however, should not only double check with the maker of the product but also get advice from their physicians.

Nuts: Almonds, hazelnuts, Brazil nuts and others, enough to fill a tablespoon, can lower bad cholesterol possibly as well as some prescription drugs if taken daily.

Fiber of Various Kinds: The type of fiber found in wheat bran and oat bran, as well as that found in beans, soy or fruit, can lower bad cholesterol by about 10% if taken daily.

Soybeans as a Protein Source: Replacing meats with soy products can lower bad cholesterol.

Chocolate: As long as you do not eat too much of it, and thus gain weight, chocolate can help to prevent heart attacks. Most of us know lots of old people who love chocolate, and they have obviously lived to tell the tale! Good chocolate contains many substances that are beneficial to health. Cocoa and chocolate are made from the beans of the cacao tree. Generally, chocolate companies do not reveal the type of cacao bean that is used in the manufacture of their products, but for your information there are two types of bean. For the highest-quality chocolate, a chocolate maker would choose Criollo or Arriba cacao beans. These high-quality beans are from a rarer Cacao tree, and are therefore more expensive to use in the manufacturing of their product. Forastero cacao beans are blended with other common beans to produce most of the chocolate found in stores and confectionery shops.

Substances called flavonoids are found in many vegetables, in tea, in red wine and in fruits. They are known to help prevent blood clots by making the blood-clotting particles, called platelets, less sticky. Chocolate, along with tea, is perhaps the best source of these flavonoids. At least one researcher, Professor Carl Keen at the University of California, has shown that chocolate is as good as aspirin in preventing blood clotting.

Good chocolate, that is, chocolate that has little or no added fat or sweetener, can be a healthy food. As long as the chocolate is a part of your diet, and not added to your food as extra calories, it should not cause weight gain, and the same is true of nuts. A health expert can help you to balance food quality and calories if you have any doubts about chocolate in your diet, and especially if you have diabetes, by suggesting the correct proportions of protein, carbohydrates, fats, vitamins and minerals.

Just like honey, chocolate is *not* bad for your teeth; in fact, they are both good for the teeth, along with cleaning and flossing. It is the fluorine in chocolate that is the most active protector, and honey has been shown to release hydrogen peroxide. Both these substances slow down the bacteria that damage teeth.

High-quality chocolate has been found to be a general stimulant and energy boost. It seems to help lift depression in some people, and it does supply the body with basic nutrients. Depending on the type of chocolate that you are eating, that is, dark, milk or white, you will be ingesting such essential substances as protein, carbohydrates, good fats, calcium, magnesium and iron, as well as various vitamins and other minerals. Theobromine, a substance similar to caffeine, is the stimulant in chocolate.

By way of ending this section, I am reminded of a real-life event from my childhood in England. I'll never forget the twin ladies who, as I was growing up, never seemed to age! Every day, they would walk down from the hills above the village, just to go to the local shop to buy their food, and then they would walk back up to their home.

I remember these twins as elderly women when I was a young boy, and yet they were still doing the same walk when I came home on breaks from university. Years after I had left England for Canada, my family and I would return for visits, only to see the selfsame twins still walking up and down the hill arm in arm!

It so happened that my youngest sister began work in that local food shop, and eventually she was able to tell me the twins' secret shopping list. For the major part of my life, these extremely fit, elderly ladies had walked an unknown number of miles every day to buy *five bars of dark chocolate and two lemons!* For all I know, they might still be walking that same route!

Illustration 10-b shows the twins, looking quite happy as they march down the long road from the hills above to the shop in the village.

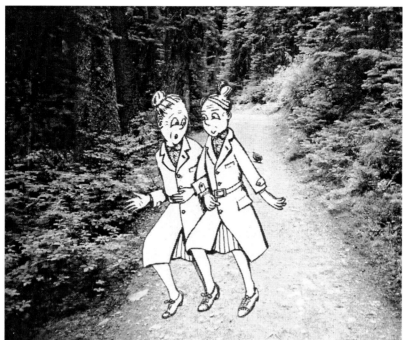

10-b These twins were seen just about every day coming down the long hilly road to the shop in the village below, but they did not seem to age from year to year. Was it their exercise or their diet or both that kept them from aging?

Vitamins that Clear Homocysteine: Vitamins B_{12}, B_6 and folic acid all help to lower the substance homocysteine in the bloodstream. In some people with raised blood levels of homocysteine, there is a higher risk of strokes, heart attacks and other blood-clotting diseases.

The vitamins that help to lower the homocysteine levels can be found in green leafy vegetables, milk, oranges, oatmeal and meats. If you are vegetarian, you can take sup-

plements of vitamin B$_{12}$ (250-500 micrograms), folic acid
(400 micrograms) and vitamin B$_6$ (25-50 milligrams).

Liquids that Are a Good Choice for the Heart

Oils: Olive oil is likely the number one vegetable source oil
that helps to lower bad cholesterol. Along with canola oil,
olive oil is rich in oleic acid, a monounsaturated and essential fatty acid. It is an essential fatty acid because it is one
that you must ingest as a food because your body cannot
make it.

Omega-6 oils are other polyunsaturated fatty acids that are
present in oils from other vegetable sources, such as the
seed oils: corn, soya, sunflower and safflower. The use of
omega-6 oils has not been proved to reduce blood-clotting-
type deaths. In fact, these compounds, with chemical structures similar to omega-3 oils, which are known to be life-
savers, could perhaps be reducing the effectiveness of the
omega-3 substances!

Tea, both black and green, has been shown to provide the
body with enough flavonoids, in the form of polyphenols,
both to lower cholesterol and reduce heart attacks. A study
from Holland has revealed that a 50% reduction in heart
attacks is possible by drinking tea. It is not known if adding
milk to tea reduces the amount of antioxidants absorbed

by the body (as it has been shown to do in chocolate). It should also be noted here that the pressed and boiled coffee that is used in some French coffees contains a substance called cafestrol. This chemical might be a factor in increasing heart attacks because it raises cholesterol.

Alcohol: Misuse of alcohol is, without a doubt, a serious health risk. If there are no health reasons why you cannot drink alcohol, moderate use can prolong life. A half to one pint of beer a day, or a small glass of brandy or red wine or the equivalent, can help to raise the good cholesterol and help to reduce the risks of a heart attack.

Too much alcohol, even once, can injure, maim or even kill you, possibly along with a friend or a family member, if you are involved in an injury of any type, and particularly in those that involve motor vehicles.

Antioxidants: Bad cholesterol, which has oxygen connected to it, is more dangerous than that same cholesterol when the oxygen has been removed. Basically, antioxidants help to stop the oxygen/cholesterol combination, thereby reducing the risks of a heart attack, or so the theory goes. Vitamin E was once thought to help stop heart attacks because of its antioxidant effect.
Studies so far have suggested that it does not work well at all to prevent such events; however, more powerful anti-

oxidants exist that do reduce heart attacks. These antioxidants occur in the form of flavonoids, and are found abundantly in teas (as noted above), in cocoa and chocolate, and in red wine. As already mentioned, regular tea drinking cuts the risk of a heart attack by 50%!

Other Ways To Lower Heart Attack Risk

Lowering cholesterol, by blocking absorption through the intestine, using various methods, can reduce the risk of a heart attack. Plant chemicals, called stanols, and sterols can reduce cholesterol levels. Some of the better margarines contain these natural compounds, although the presence of trans-fatty acids would render these foods harmful.

Good and bad cholesterol are made in the liver, as are triglycerides (fats). Helping the liver to make more good cholesterol and less bad cholesterol/triglycerides is another way to lessen heart attack rates.
Moderate exercise, prescribed medications, and the vitamin niacin can all be used to help the liver to do a good job!

So, if you can shed stress, exercise, control your blood pressure to a normal level, stop smoking and avoid secondhand cigarette smoke, control any diabetes, keep to a perfect weight, that is, check that your waist circumference is normal, and eat and drink the perfect 'fuel' for your body, you will not die young of a heart attack.

Before looking at cancers and diet, let us look at the bioflavonoids and list them, because their names are not only confusing but also similarly spelled. Adding to the confusion is that some terms are spelled in a variety of ways. For example, "flavonoid" is sometimes spelled "flavinoid," and sometimes "flavanoid." They all mean the same thing. For clarity's sake, the first spelling will be used here.

There are at least twenty types of bioflavonoids (flavonoids). The common names that you will see listed in health articles are as follows:

Flavones	Isoflavones	Flavonols
Flavonones	Polyphenols	Rutin
Catechins	d-Limonene	Nobiletin
Quercetin	Naringin	Tangeretin

Generally, they all act as antioxidants, substances that clear harmful chemicals called free radicals from the body. Bioflavonoids are also able to clear allergy-causing substances from the body, as well as other bad chemicals that cause inflammation.

Food and Cancers

Doctors and scientists have known for years that many cancers are caused by substances that enter our bodies one way or another. It has also been known, and for just as long, that other substances that we eat can help to stop the formation of cancers.

It took time for us to realize it, but eventually we came to understand that factory workers who handled aniline dyes stood a high chance of getting bladder cancer. Asbestos, if breathed into the lungs, was found to be one of the causes of mesothelioma, that is, a type of cancer of the lung surface.

Many lists are available from the many cancer organizations of known and suspected substances that can cause cancer. These can often be found on websites, using the "cancer" search term. Despite the extensive research for more information on cancer-causing agents, there are still many common cancers that cannot be explained.

Breast and colon cancers continue to be common, and not fully controlled, types of new growths. The causes of these two cancers have yet to be found. Since the 1950s, colon cancer has been associated with eating beef, and studies carried out since that time have continued to suggest that beef is a factor. Many causes for breast cancer have been suggested: underarm deodorants/antiperspirants, viruses, obesity factors, breast cancer genes, alcohol, exposure to light during the sleeping hours, insecticides in food, x-rays (a mammogram, as I have already warned you, gives out one thousand times more radiation than a chest x-ray), and perhaps acrylamides.

Often when a cause is found for a cancer, until it has been proved time and time again, there is a tendency for the public — and some doctors — to ignore the possibility of that finding being true. Over the years, there have been many false alarms of substances being accused of causing cancers. Time and research eventually give us accurate answers to the many claims of cancer causes. There is no doubt, however, that smoking cigarettes for a prolonged period can cause lung cancer, along with cancer of the larynx and of the bladder. Nor should secondhand smoke from cigarettes be forgotten as a cause for disease, definitely contributing to both lung cancer and heart disease. Asbestos has been mentioned already as a known cause for mesothelioma, a deadly type of lung cancer. Viruses can also cause some cancers. Liver cancer (hepatocellular carcinoma), for instance, can be caused by the hepatitis B virus, and cancer of the neck of the womb (cervix) by the cause of the common wart, that is, human papilloma virus (HPV). These facts might be somewhat oversimplified, in that the viruses might have to have other factors present to do their dirty work. An example would be where a woman who smokes regularly, and has an HPV-infected cervix, would have a higher risk of cancer of the cervix than a woman who had just HPV.

For more information on cancer causes, such as environmental factors, see the websites of the many cancer organizations that publish excellent fact sheets on this topic.

Colon cancer, along with lung cancer, is the second most common cause for death in the world. As with many cancers, the cause for colon cancer is likely a mixture of factors. The known facts on colon cancer triggers, or suspicious reasons for getting it, include the following:

Not enough exercise (or perhaps, conversely, excessive exercise);

Lack of fruits and vegetables (lack of flavonoids);

Too little selenium in the diet;

Beef, especially barbecued or roasted for various reasons;

Baked or deep-fried food and Chlorine in water (10% of

colon and bladder cancers could be caused by this).

Acrylamides have caused quite a stir in the scientific community. In some countries, this substance is used in water treatment to help filter off particles in the drinking water. These acrylamides have been studied for human and animal safety and have demonstrated a definite health hazard. Long-term exposure has been shown to cause nervous system disorders and cancers. In 2002, scientific researchers in Sweden and in the United Kingdom announced an extremely significant discovery. They found that many everyday foods, ones that were clear of contaminants before baking or frying, contained a large amount of acrylamides after they had been baked or deep fried. Everyday foods such as french fries, packaged chips, bread, beef, and many other baked and deep-fried foods contained acrylamide amounts well above the safety levels calculated for drinking water! Despite this, many health authorities have advised the public not to worry yet about the findings, stating that a known toxin, even though it has now been discovered to be present in certain common foods, should not be reduced in their diets until further notice! Acrylamides *are* dangerous, and the ingesting or eating of these substances should be reduced to a minimum.

Selenium has been found to help prevent colon cancer, along with other cancers and blood-clotting diseases. In one study, the trial was stopped early because it was quite obvious that the people taking selenium were not getting colon cancer, whereas the non-selenium-takers were getting colon cancer at the normal rate.

Many foods contain selenium, ranging from fish (no surprise), broccoli (can be high or low, depending on the soil it has been grown in), nuts (especially Brazil nuts), and wheat germ to brewer's yeast. Some studies show that the form of selenium synthesized in plants, such as broccoli, has a better cancer-preventing action than the types put into tablet form. The tablet form of selenium uses a salt form called selenium selenite, or selenate. This salt form of selenium can prevent cancers, but the person taking it should be careful not to take too much, because toxicity is possible. Broccoli contains a form of selenium called selenium methyl seleno-cysteine, which will not be toxic if you overdose on this "king" of all vegetables.

An American study (in Iowa) found that tea drinkers suffered less cancer of the bladder, kidneys and bowel. Catechin, another antioxidant in tea, might be the anti-cancer substance that protects our bodies from the many pro-cancer chemicals.

What then is the right way to eat? It sounds so complicated to avoid saturated fats, to avoid acrylamides (frying and baking are bad), to eat flavonoids of the correct type, to avoid chlorine, to avoid beef, and yet manage to eat products from the food guides to stay healthy!

If we look back to the beginning of this topic of good body "fuel", and remind ourselves which type of eating really works at prolonging life, then we come to a simple solution to the question of why do Cretan and Japanese women — the longevity champions of the world — avoid an early death so well.

Being physically fit, not smoking and avoiding secondhand smoke, and eating in a healthy way, as shown above, along with avoiding injuries, could certainly reduce considerably your chances of dying earlier than necessary. If Japanese women live longer than all other women because they naturally eat well and are fitter than average, we should all be able to learn from them.

For a summary of healthy foods, please refer to the tables that follow. These directions are not a complete manual on nutrition but will hopefully help you think before you eat. If food is safe to eat raw then ingest it in the natural state, otherwise, boiling or steaming are healthy ways to prepare the meal.

A Way To Eat To Live Longer by Avoiding Heart Attacks and Cancer

Food Type	Reason for Eating
Eat a variety of *fish*, three to five times a week. Steamed or poached is the healthiest way to cook this proven health food. Avoid farmed salmon if possible because the wild variety is the safest.	A study published in an April 2002 edition of the American Medical Association, called "The Nurses' Health Study," revealed that eating fish seemed to reduce substantially the risk of both developing heart disease and dying from it. Moreover, those women who ate the higher quantity of fish also had the lowest death rate. There have been other studies that also reveal that eating fish prolongs life.
Consume greens and other *fruits* and *vegetables*. A variety of colors is appetizing and is good for your health. Try to eat six to ten portions a day.	This part of your diet provides minerals, vitamins, fiber and *flavonoids*. Most flavonoids are antioxidants, some are "anti" other bad chemicals in the body, and different types are known to help prevent heart disease and cancers. Include a source of selenium, eg, broccoli.

Food Type	Reason for Eating
Eat lots of *fiber:* bran, psyllium, fruits and vegetables.	Lowering bad cholesterol can help to reduce a heart attack. Pushing cancer-causing substances quickly through the bowel reduces the colon cancer risk.
Avoid saturated fats and over-cooked foods as much as possible: Roast beef, deep-fried potatoes and other barbecued foods. In fact, many baked foods form acrylamides, which is felt to be one of the causes of some common cancers. Beef fat has been shown to be a part cause, at least, of prostate cancer.	*No reason for eating* unless these foods are your only choice. Essential fats, oils, amino acids, vitamins and minerals are all provided by the recommended foods.
Better quality chocolate (unless you have a medical condition that says otherwise).	The flavonoids in high-quality chocolate can be as good as aspirin in preventing strokes and heart attacks. (Note also that aspirin has been shown to reduce the risk of colon cancer.)

Food Type	Reason for Eating
Alcohol, in the form of red wine, brandy and beer, can be healthy in small quantities, as long as your liver and stomach are not diseased. Your own physician should advise. Generally, two drinks daily can be safe (equivalent to two small beers).	Red wine contains good flavonoids, and alcohol generally raises the good cholesterol. Too much alcohol is damaging to the heart; small amounts are good for it. Heavy drinking appears to be another cause for colon polyps and cancer.
Black or green *tea* seemingly reduces both heart attack rates and bladder, bowel and kidney cancers.	*Polyphenols* (flavonoids) are antioxidants and can protect our arteries from damage. *Catechins* in tea have an anti-cancer effect.

A note on balance should be the final word here. Because foods that might be thought of as unhealthy can still be part of a diet plan as long as other chosen fuels have anti-disease properties. Desserts, for example, can be used as long as the total daily calorie intake is not exceeded. If those tasty foods contain flavonoids, have lots of fiber, and are low in bad fats and calories, then including them as part of a healthy diet is to be encouraged. When trying to avoid diseases, we should also be trying to enjoy life which can include tasty treats!

Chapter 11

A Few More Ways To Kill Yourself

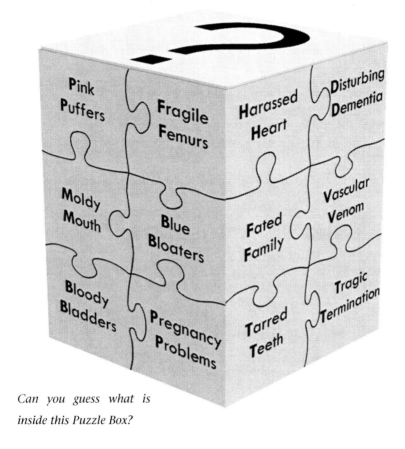

Can you guess what is inside this Puzzle Box?

Many people do not follow doctors' orders. This situation is called *non-compliance*. Even doctors themselves are guilty of this act when they are given medical advice.

It is curious that many patients who have had opportunities to avoid suffering and death continue to insult their bodies anyway, knowing full well that they will end up an ugly sight or a disfigured person, or even die younger than they should. Most of these people are unaware that they are already silently ill. They are not necessarily "suicidal" either, but likely it is that they think that they will be an exception to the normal occurrence and not suffer the results of body self-abuse.

We have all heard the comment, "We have all got to die of something!" Unfortunately, this declaration is made by many who have a built-in excuse for doing something that they know is destructive to their bodies. They give themselves permission to continue their suicidal mission. Would the average non-suicidal human lie down on a busy freeway or motorway for a rest, knowing that they would be crushed to death? "No" is the obvious answer to this odd question, but every day there are many who perform slow versions of an *equivalent action*, destroying themselves, cell by cell, until their major organs are severely damaged or until they expire in a miserable way.

How do you kill yourself or make yourself suffer in ways often worse than a crushing crash to the ground?

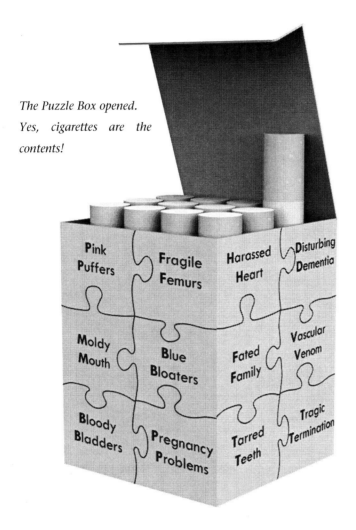

The Puzzle Box opened.
Yes, cigarettes are the
contents!

Pink Puffers

Fragile Femurs

Harassed Heart

Disturbing Dementia

Moldy Mouth

Blue Bloaters

Fated Family

Vascular Venom

Bloody Bladders

Pregnancy Problems

Tarred Teeth

Tragic Termination

The puzzle box shown here will reveal to you one of the most direct causes of a self-destruction process; you will see that it is *smoking cigarettes.*

Every day that a smoker inhales cigarette smoke, or innocent non-smokers breathe in those same fumes, the cells in their various organs struggle. These tiny, delicate units of life have to overcome the effects of the toxins that are introduced into the organs that they make up. Many of these cells have more lives than a cat, but they eventually give up and die, or at least change to adapt to the many tarry chemicals that they have to bathe in. It is these cells that change their shape that eventually turn into cancers.

Many smokers think that the damage to their bodies takes many years to develop. Every time a smoker inhales, however, there are *immediate* effects, as well as the buildup of the groundwork for the slower, long-term diseases. Two examples of immediate body changes are an almost instant reduction in blood flow to a variety of organs, such as the uterus in a pregnant woman or the heart muscle in anyone, and immediate stomach bleeding, which is seen in some people following a drag on a cigarette.

Who are these smokers of the world?

Some women feel that cigarettes help to keep them slim, and others smoke to relieve stress or boredom. Strong addiction to nicotine keeps people puffing, and this is an unfortunate situation for those with imminently life-threatening diseases, because, even when they have a chance to save themselves, they just cannot stop smoking.

This is an extremely sad time for a family and doctor to witness.

Looking at the puzzle box, and particularly at the conditions on the pieces, I wonder how many diseases you, the reader, recognized as being a part of smoking.

Here are the answers to the puzzle box pieces:

Pink Puffers: This refers to emphysema, a lung disease where the air spaces at the end of each bronchial tube are enlarged and damaged, thus reducing the total surface area of membrane that can absorb oxygen. Most people with this disease are smokers, are short of breath, and tend to be pinkish in appearance and to puff as they breathe through pursed lips. They are not blue around the lips unless the emphysema is extremely bad.

Moldy Mouth: This is the unmistakable odor that other people can smell coming from the mouth of a person who smokes cigarettes when that unfortunate person speaks. This condition is hard to cover up; the only treatment is to totally stop the habit.

Bloody Bladders: Heavy bleeding into the bladder has to be tested extensively by a doctor. Blood in the urine has many causes, one being bladder cancer. Some bladder cancers are caused by, yes, cigarette smoking.

Fragile Femurs: An easily broken thigh bone occurs with osteoporosis, which was described in the chapters on that disease. At the closest point to the hip, the femur bone forms the ball of the hip joint, and it is just below this region that the bone is most fragile in osteoporosis. A fracture here is a serious complication of a fall. Cigarette smoking is a factor that can cause osteoporosis because it is a daily bone cell toxin; however, it can be removed from the blood stream just by stopping the inhalation of tobacco fumes.

Blue Bloaters: Chronic bronchitis is a disease of the tubes of the lung structures where the lining cells are damaged by air pollution, smoking, and other chemicals that are breathed into the airways. A cough, shortness of breath, and coughing up phlegm are common symptoms. It is not unusual for the sufferer to have a slightly dusky or blue appearance, and the face starts to look blown out or bloated because breathing out takes a longer than average time. This blue-bloated condition, if allowed to continue, will combine with emphysema to become chronic obstructive pulmonary disease (COPD).

Pregnancy Problems: Smoking cigarettes in pregnancy is known to reduce the blood flow to the unborn child. As noted above, it cuts that vital supply of nutrients and oxygen immediately with each inhalation of poisonous vapor. The development of the affected baby is slowed, causing low weight and the risk of unnecessary complications at birth.

Harassed Heart: Cigarette smoke contains pro-oxidants, substances that help to build known noxious free radicals. The addition of oxygen to some natural chemicals in the body causes that presumably safe substance to turn into a dangerous one. Bad cholesterol, for example, is a lot more damaging when oxygen is combined with it; and tobacco substances are great at ensuring this dangerous union.

Within seconds of inhaling cigarette smoke, coronary arteries narrow spasmodically. Additionally, the chemicals inhaled allow the cholesterol to become more damaging to the artery linings. This creates the perfect setup for a heart attack!

Fated Family: People who smoke cigarettes reduce their life expectancy, and this is well-known to insurance companies. Unfortunately, it is not only the patient with the smoker's disease who suffers the misery but also the relatives, friends and health care workers who must watch that person deteriorate and slowly die.

Tarred Teeth: A regular woman smoker, even of filtered cigarettes, must work hard to keep those brown tarry deposits from building up in layers on the teeth and ruining her cosmetic appearance.

Disturbing Dementia: In the same way that cigarette smoke acts as a pro-oxidant and damages the arteries of the heart, it can also affect those vessels that supply the brain. If the blood supply is reduced to the brain, obviously serious conditions will develop. Loss of memory, associated with what is called vascular dementia, and strokes are just two diseases that lead to nasty complications.

Vascular Venom: This term refers to the damage to the arterial lining, or endothelium, that occurs when tobacco products are inhaled through the lungs and absorbed into the bloodstream. Nicotine and tar products are the culprits, so people have to avoid smokers and smoking.

Tragic Termination: Early death can be a blessing to many sufferers of smoking-related disease. Dying of lung failure is one of the most unpleasant ways to pass on from the land of the living. Lung, throat and bladder cancers, as everyone knows because they are so common, are killers that offer much suffering. Strokes and heart attacks, gangrene of the feet, and eye disease are certainly listed as well, because they change everyone's life — forever.

This description of smoker's disease is not meant to be complete, because there are a lot more features that could be described. The major point is that everyone has to keep away from tobacco products if they care about their loved ones and about their own safety.

How can a person stop smoking? This is always the common question from those who are considering breaking this self-destructive habit. After all, smokers age quickly, because the facial skin loses its youthful glow, and they get oodles of diseases to go with that "old" look.

There are many cancer clinics and other health departments that offer help to support a person's wish to break away from the grip of the mighty cigarette monster. Beginning by visiting a qualified health practitioner is always an excellent way to start the process of reducing disease risks. A combination of methods is a good way to be successful with the first try. But if one method fails, brace yourself, and try again, because eventually one treatment or another will work for you.

Smoking cessation has been seen to be achieved with some of the following methods.

- Simple discussions with an anti-smoking friend or expert.

- Hypnosis by a therapist with expertise in nicotine addiction.

- Psychological methods, using relaxation and anger management, help with marriage and other social issues. If the therapist works with cigarette addiction, advice on the many ways to break bad habits, using behavioral therapy and biofeedback, can work in certain cases.

- The use of special computer aids; progressively stronger cigarette filters, which weaken the amount of nicotine inhaled by the person needing help; and substitute cigarettes, including the type that use the marshmallow plant, and many other plant products, have all helped some smokers.

- Nicotine patches, which dispense gradually reduced levels of nicotine into the bloodstream, help to break the craving for a smoke.

- A consultation with the person's physician is often necessary for their own methods to be tried, along with a prescription perhaps to help with any identified disease that needs treatment.

Medications that help could include bupropion, which

raises the level of dopamine in the brain, a natural che-mical also stimulated by nicotine.

If a woman's body fat is the concern, in that she is worried that the cessation of smoking will cause her to gain weight, then diet, exercise and, if needed, medication for any excess abdominal girth will have to be prescribed.

If even one person is able to stop smoking cigarettes because of reading this chapter, then it will have been worth the effort of spending an entire day in preparing this relatively small amount of information on a dreadfully serious health risk.

After almost thirty years of medical practice experience, one of the greatest rewards a doctor can receive is to see a patient stop smoking, to be able to watch them appreciate the new feeling of good health, and to see them live!

Saving lives by preventing injuries was the original purpose of this project, but teaching them landing reflexes is not going to help a person dying from lung cancer. *If you smoke anything, please stop! Save your cells ... and perhaps your life as well!*

Chapter 12

How Can I Help You?

If you feel dragged down, suffer extreme tiredness, or feel, as some people put it, like a solid lump of lead, with no energy at all, it is essential for you to read the information below.

Does the average person know what goes on behind the closed doors of a doctor's examining room? Obviously, they do not; only the patients themselves and their doctor really knows the words spoken and the examination performed. As a doctor, I can certainly talk about some of the things I experience from day to day, which will be of great importance to some of those people who are reading this particular chapter. I will not, of course, be describing any of my patient's private medical files.

Let me describe some typical situations in my average day. I am going to exclude those that this whole book is about, namely injuries, and the filling out of forms for insurance companies and similar organizations, as well as common, non-serious virus infections, routine normal examinations, minor skin disorders, and other disorders not listed below.

This is not a medical textbook of diseases, but I do have to discuss, at the least, the following conditions that can weaken you to the point where a fall could occur, which can then lead to severe and even permanent damage to your health.

It is interesting to note that these reasons are similar to those given as to why people cannot, or do not, exercise.

Please look at this list. Would you answer "yes" to any them?

1)   Are you absolutely *exhausted*? That is you cannot get enough sleep to relieve your extreme tiredness, and no amount of rest will dispel your symptoms.

2)   Do you have persistent *pain* anywhere? This could include headaches, muscle pain, joint/low back pain, and skin burning, abdominal or pelvic pain.

3)   Are you *dizzy*?

4) Is your body *weight* a problem? *Excess body fat* is an extremely common problem.

5)   How is your mood? Do you feel nervous, or anxious? Do you experience panic attacks, or perhaps suffer from *persistent depression*?

There are other medical complaints that could have been listed here as well.

But for the five groups of disorders listed above, there are two common facts that connect them: they are all common, and they can all increase the risk of a fall injury. These conditions are not always easy to diagnose, and even when we know the answer to the problem they are not easy to treat. So, if you did answer "yes" to any of the five problems, you should find the information below extremely interesting!

Persistent Tiredness

There are whole books written about this subject, because the causes of tiredness and weakness are so extensive. As with all chronic medical complaints, a detailed discussion or history of the problem, as well as a thorough physical examination and tests, have to be carried out on the person who is feeling extremely tired.

Descriptions of fatigue do not vary a lot between people. Absolute exhaustion, feeling weak, and being drained of energy are some of the more familiar descriptions I hear when a person is upset enough to come to me to ask for help with the symptoms of prolonged tiredness.

An easy way to understand some of the causes for the miserable feeling of extreme, persistent fatigue is to study the diagram of the yawning lady, who is on her way to her afternoon job, but still tired despite a good night's sleep and a restful morning (see illustration 12-a).

Illustration 12-a Some of the many reasons why you could be tired

Depression, worry/anxiety/sleep disorders

Muscle disease (myositis)

Various types of anemia (iron, B_{12} lack, genetic, and many other types)

Allergies (Candida/yeasts)

Obesity

Medications (drugs)

Chronic poisonings

Intestinal parasites

Cancer (hidden types)

Autoimmune (lupus, rheumatoid arthritis, and many other similar diseases)

Diabetes or low blood sugar addictions (alcohol/drugs)

Multiple sclerosis and other nervous system disorders (myasthenia gravis)

Thyroid disorders (low or high)
Chronic infections (TB, kidney infections, mononucleosis, HIV, hepatitis, Lyme disease, etc)

Menopause or andropause

Chronic organ disease (kidney failure, lung, liver or heart*)

Adrenal gland disease

Chronic fatigue syndrome Fibromyalgia (fibrositis)

Herb/drug reactions

Mineral deficiencies (eg, zinc)

[*Variation of angina]

Some of the medical problems shown are not common, but they are listed because they might help a reader who suffers from fatigue to find the cause of their symptoms.

Remember, or at least realize, rare conditions do occur, and it could be you, the reader, who has a rare cause for the tiredness.

When being assessed for a diagnosis for whatever problem you suffer, you have to realize that most patients seen in an average doctor's day do not have a serious condition. A skill that needs to be sharpened by all us doctors is to be able to pick out those people with the rare, serious conditions among the common not-so-serious disorders.

One common cause of ill health is heart disease caused by blocked coronary arteries, as well it is a common cause for dying early. Many women who start with angina do not always have the typical chest pain that is described in many medical articles. One of the atypical symptoms of angina is persistent tiredness. If blood tests cannot find a cause for you becoming *easily exhausted*, it is a good idea to get some heart tests done.

If you think you have identified a cause for your feelings of severe tiredness, discuss the possibility with *your doctor*. If you have another source of medical help, you will obviously seek the alternative care as well, but please get any serious conditions screened first because they might be time sensitive. Many cancers, for example, can be cured if caught early.

Disagreement does exist among doctors, not only on the treatment of certain diseases but also on the very existence of some others. One example is the yeast allergy condition. It is well-known that yeast infections cause mouth or vaginal irritations, and that yeasts can invade other areas of your body, such as the gullet, skin or throat, if you are suffering from a disease where your immune system is weakened.

A sensitivity to Candida albicans, as shown by a skin allergy test, in my experience does exist as a cause for persistent ill health. This condition might not be a super-common cause; however, if a patient suffers malaise, fatigue, abdominal pain or other chronic symptoms that are not explained by any other tests or examinations, then a test for this yeast sensitivity should be ordered. If the test is positive, the treatment given is called immunotherapy. This treatment consists of a series of injections, similar to allergy injections, with an extract of Candida albicans. If this treatment is the correct choice, it should be effective, at least partly, within two months.

Rarely, it is worth checking for arsenic, or selenium or similar poisons in the blood as a cause for not feeling well. Otherwise, use the diagram as a checklist for fatigue causes.

There is one doctor's comment that a person does not want to hear, and that is this:

"Your medical examination is normal, and all your tests are normal, so I have no idea what is causing your severe tiredness; therefore, I cannot offer any treatment."

Worse than this comment is this:

"Your tests are normal, but you are a woman, so you will just have to go home and try to get over it."

What does a desperately tired woman do in this situation?

Because fatigue is common and a significant risk in fall injuries, each person disabled by this problem has to be treated. Before looking at possible remedies, a list of reasons as to why a diagnosis is often not made follows.

1) Because of the high cost of tests, the doctor who ordered them might not have done every test possible that could detect the rare causes for fatigue. It is important to discuss this with the doctor, because sometimes it is a factor that hinders a diagnosis.

2) Even if all tests are carried out, it is quite possible that no test exists that will ever reveal the true cause of your

disorder. Having said this, medical tests can at least exclude other causes for your symptoms.

3) In the case of severe tiredness, and when the cause has not been found, it might be necessary for you to be referred to a doctor who either specializes or at least has a special interest in fatigue. Your health practitioner can arrange this for you.

4) What to do when all else fails? For example, you are tired, and all tests and specialists cannot find a reason why you are suffering. Some people in this situation take a variety of herbal/mineral supplements, or perhaps participate in ancient exercise systems, or seek help from the numerous complementary therapists available. Multitudes of both trained and untrained people offer many treatments for anyone with almost any chronic health condition that does not respond to traditional therapy, and sometimes even as a first treatment as well. I have seen many useful, safe treatments, but I have also seen some dishonest, unsafe and expensive remedies given to desperate people.

One treatment that is worth trying is a course of vitamin B_{12} injections. Blood levels of this vitamin should be checked, of course, in the tests done as part of your medical examination, but studies done on patients with Alzheimer's disease and other memory disorders have found that these patients benefit from extra B_{12}, even when their level is normal.

Any test has a range of normal for, say, a blood level of a chemical. An upper and a lower level are usually listed on the laboratory results form. These tests can be interpreted in different ways. If they are interpreted too strictly, it can be possible to let some people with a disease have a diagnosis missed.

Sometimes a blood level of a chemical for one person needs to be at a quite different level for another person to have the same effect in the way that they feel. Here are a few chemical examples: thyroid, vitamin B_{12} and even hemoglobin. It is not a rare occasion for laboratories to change their ranges of normal to match other more up-to-date laboratories.

Even using the same units, normal levels can vary for a test between different blood-testing facilities. At the present time, to be considered abnormal for a TSH thyroid test, and using the same units, one laboratory has a level of 4 listed as a maximum, another claims that the level has to be 9. It is too bad if your level is 8 at the one center, because you will be told that there is nothing wrong with you! If the level 4 is used as a guide, and the patient is treated based on that level being the normal level, symptoms usually improve.

The message here is this: Ask questions about your tests, and find out just what the *average* blood levels are. It is sometimes not good enough to be *just* scraping into the normal range.

Now, getting back to B_{12} treatment, many blood test results forms state that a deficiency of vitamin B_{12} exists if the levels are less than the number 150 units; this is partly true, but this also means that a person has to have a blood level below this number to be recognized as suffering a deficiency, that is, low enough to cause serious disease. What happens if you are just above this level? I can tell you the answer. Most people are told that they do not have a problem with a low vitamin B_{12}! Let me put this idea another way. If your B_{12} is 151 units, technically you have a normal B_{12}; however if that level is 149 units, then your level would be recorded as being low, and treatment would be offered. So, long before your B_{12} gets to the magical 150 level, you will certainly have symptoms of that essential substance dropping, namely fatigue!

Disability insurance companies, along with other similar organizations, often do not recognize pain as a disability, in much the same way as medical testing facilities do not always consider tiredness to be a problem, thus there is no level listed as to what level of B_{12} causes fatigue! The same is true of thyroid, iron and other necessary blood levels of essential substances. By the way, the level of B_{12} that I feel is necessary to be average and not tired is a level of 300 units plus; moreover, in almost thirty years of giving some people as high as 3000 units of B_{12}, I have never seen a side effect — but I have definitely seen lots of good effects!

One remedy that does not need a medical test before trying as a therapy for weariness/extreme tiredness is the amino acid called tryptophan. In most countries, tryptophan is now a prescribed natural food substance, with the dose that can help being about 750mg once or twice a day. In some people, tryptophan is so effective that it can cause insomnia if taken too late in the evening. Obviously, a medical practitioner has to supervise anyone taking it to monitor the effectiveness and any side effects, and to check, of course, that another treatable disease is not the cause for the severe fatigue.

Of course, there have been many other remedies used for fatigue by various health practitioners over time, including stimulant tonics (containing substances such as pipradol), zinc, extra natural thyroid, etc, but some carry with them the risk of long-term side effects. The health practitioner who knows you the best is the most suitable person to consult if you suffer from fatigue.

Just remember, *if you are tired*, even for short periods, *at least try to avoid an injury.*

Pain

At one time or another, everyone experiences some sort of pain, but that pain is a serious problem if it goes on from day to day. We are talking about pain that we know the cause of, pain that is hard to diagnose, and pain that is hard to treat. Whatever aspect of pain we look at, apart from making one miserable, it does affect a person's concentration, often to the point where it can lead to a risk of injury.

Chronic pain can be caused by cancers; arthritis; previous, as well as current, injuries; muscle disease; chronic strain injuries, including the neck, the low back, and other joints; migraine and other headaches; bone disease; dental or jaw disorders; sinusitis; angina, as well as other diseases of the arteries, including those of the legs; complications of diabetes; diseases of the nervous system; ingrown toenails; and intestinal pain. The list, of course, can go on and on with many other causes.

With pain that is hard to diagnose, many opinions might have to be sought. If your health practitioner finds it difficult to identify the cause of your pain, you could well need a referral to a doctor who has an interest in so-called *difficult diagnoses*, as well as in pain control. Most cities have a pain clinic, where experts in pain control are available for consultation.

Important Fact — All medical tests are *not* 100% accurate. This includes all x-rays (mammograms included), ultrasounds, and even MRIs! Yes, Magnetic Resonance Imaging can miss disease for at least two reasons.

Reason 1: It cannot distinguish normal from abnormal organ tissue.

Reason 2: The specialist who interprets the MRI films does not see the abnormality for one reason or another.

Sometimes the diagnosis of fibromyalgia is made, which is only serious because, at the time of writing, there is no cure. It is always important to make sure that there is not a hidden cancer causing persistent pain.

Whether the cause for the pain is known or not, it is important to control this miserable symptom. Depending on the type of pain you have, there are a variety of pain control methods available. The list is long, and includes various medications, physical methods (physiotherapy, massage therapy, acupuncture, TENS, other electrical stimulators, Shiatzu, etc), hypnosis and herbal therapies. Just simply talking to an expert about the pain can help.

As mentioned above, there are many clinics that specialize in pain control, but obviously it is extremely important to find the reason for the pain and to treat that cause.

Dizziness

This, of course, is a major problem as a direct cause for falling injuries. It is just as important to cure the cause as to control the symptoms. To diagnose prolonged dizziness/vertigo/loss of balance, a specialist in neurology or ear disorders is almost always needed. If you are interested in all the causes for dizziness, you will have to understand the workings of the inner ear; the brain, including the cerebellum; the blood supply to the brain; the effects of drugs or alcohol on blood pressure and the brain; as well as general diseases that affect balance (see the chapter that discusses the *balance point*).

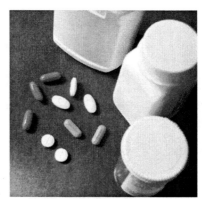

12-b Various tablets as a possible cause for dizzy spells

Photograph 12-b is a reminder that some prescribed, as well as off-the-shelf medications, can be responsible for dizziness or light-headedness.

Vertigo has to be diagnosed, and it should not be confused with general dizziness. Often, with vertigo, you feel as if you are spinning/rotating, and nausea is a common symptom associated with the inability to control balance.

Tests ordered include blood tests, an MRI, and a test called an ENG, but not until a thorough physical examination has been carried out. Once the cause for the dizziness is found, the disease can be treated if it is possible to do so.

Incurable dizziness does occur, however, and so there are various medications, as well as exercises, that can be given to the patient who suffers from this annoying and definitely disabling condition.

In rare cases, an operation is needed either on the brain or on part of the inner sections of the ear.

See your doctor if you suffer from vertigo or general dizziness. If a definite diagnosis cannot be reached though, you should consider a referral to a specialized ear clinic, because the problem might have a simple solution.

Is Losing Weight Your Problem?

It shapes

It pads

It insulates

It can be sensuous

It can be upsetting

It can be a health risk

It is also a storage organ

It is, naturally, fat!

Although body fat can to some extent protect your bones from the impact of a fall, the excess weight can increase the force of the fall. Generally, being overweight can decrease the chance of a hip fracture but increase the chance of an ankle fracture, according to several studies, from countries such as Finland (OSTPRE, published in *Bone*, 2002), and the United Kingdom (published in *Injury*, 1996).

The problem of excess body fat is a worsening one for most of the civilized world, and what is truly alarming is that more than half the population are affected.

It is interesting that, although being fat is more common in men, it is women who seek help the most to lose their excess weight. This problem, called *obesity* by us health practitioners, is thought by some to be a disease, but other doctors and scientists refute this classification.

In recent times, much scientific evidence has been produced to suggest why some people gain weight — and cannot lose it — and why some people's appetites are so insatiable. All the details of the scientific evidence cannot be given here, because it would take the whole book to write about this interesting and important topic; however, there are a few important facts that have to be noted.

Some people who are overweight are that way because they have big appetites. It is upsetting for these people to be this way, but even more so when they are called greedy, or are told that it is their fault that they are fat simply because they eat too much. Comments from health professionals, such as, "If you eat less, you will lose weight," do little to help most patients with large appetites. It is likely that most doctors have seen the cartoon in one of the medical journals that shows a fat, frustrated patient asking the doctor, "Why is it that, after five years of medical training, the only advice you can give me to lose weight is to eat less." Patients do expect more from their doctors and indeed all professionals.

It is hoped that it is some relief for those with big appetites to know that medical scientists have found a small number of chemicals in the body that control appetite. It is these chemicals that go out of balance, causing in turn an increase in the appetite. One chemical, a hormone found in fat cells, is called Leptin, and for unknown reasons it stops doing its proper job on an area of the brain called the hypothalamus. Gut hormones can lose their appetite control on the brain as well, and there are other hormone-type chemicals that affect appetite, which will be named as soon as the research is complete. At the time of compiling this information, for those of you with a scientific interest in excess body fat, at least two stomach hormones have been discovered that control the appetite or fat content of the body: one is called Ghrelin (discovered by Japanese scientists in 1999) and the other is Cholecystokinin, a well-known substance that was found to have an effect on appetite only in recent years.

Make sure that your feelings of hunger are not simply too much stomach acid, or some other intestinal problem. There is actually a long list of medical reasons why an appetite can be strong: stress, depression, low self-esteem and excess alcohol intake are just some of the causes. All can be explained though by the way these medical disorders cause an effect on the hypothalamus region of the brain.

Obesity, apart from being associated with inactivity, is known to be partly genetic. It seems that some fat people are born with enzymes that make more fat than those in slim people.

Now, on the subject of slim people, extra thin people are as difficult to treat as fat people. Most doctors will have a patient in their practice who, despite eating huge amounts of food, cannot gain weight. Do these opposite type of people have a reverse chemical problem to fat people? I do not know, and I have never seen a study on this *skinny* problem.

Every health practitioner involved with helping obese people has patients who, despite low-calorie diets and exercise, still cannot lose weight. In most cases, this is due to chemical imbalances. How do doctors help these patients? First of all, the body fat is assessed by the body mass index (BMI), fat percentage, waist measurement, or other methods. *If* obesity is diagnosed, then a history of the problem (family risks of obesity/diseases, drugs/alcohol, when and how the weight problem started, etc) is discussed, and a physical examination is done. Blood tests should be carried out, along with other necessary tests, such as an ECG, before treatment is started.

If a cause is not found for the person's weight problem, then the quantity and quality of the food intake has to be assessed and the amount of physical activity has to be looked at. The health practitioner can then recommend treatment by way of food changes and exercise methods.

Many excellent — as well as not so excellent — ways to eat to lose weight exist, and regularly we hear about a new diet that is *better than all others*. This book is not designed to discuss all these diets, but certain ideas are common to some of these eating methods, and certainly can work if they are followed accurately. Here are some of the features of the general principles that can help in body fat control:

1) Have breakfast every day.

2) When trying to lose excess body fat, keep to about one starch serving a day, less than 30% fat (30% of total calories) and have lots of protein (first class, such as fish, as well as second class, such as lots of beans).

3) Snack bars designed to help weight control can be used if they are substituted into the diet plan.

4) Maintenance of body weight can be achieved with three starch servings, again less than 30% fat, and the balance of the calories in proteins. Your total calorie needs will, of course, depend on your energy needs for each day, which

presumably will vary from day to day and depend on the season.

5) Appetite control is usually a problem, and antacids, water, sucking a lemon, and eating low calorie foods, such as cucumbers, can all help. In selected people, an appetite suppressant medication can be used. Try to avoid sweet foods such as cake, candy and sugar, and replace them with more proteins, for example, fish, poultry, low fat cheese, beans, peas and lentils.

The type of exercise recommended varies according to a person's health, but generally aerobic activity works better than resistance exercises, at least for weight control. It is useful to know how many calories are used for different activities, so some examples follow:

Walking slowly at a steady pace (2.5 mph/4 kmh) uses 200 calories.

Walking briskly (3-4 mph/5-6.5 kmh) uses 300 calories.

Cycling uses 250-1000 calories per hour.

Swimming uses 400-900 calories per hour.

Tennis uses 450-750 calories per hour.

Running (jogging at 4.5-8.0 mph/7-13 kmh) uses 450 plus calories, depending on wind direction and temperature, and on whether you are running on hills or flat ground. Walking and running with a dog is an excellent way to keep fit as well as lose pounds of fat (see photograph 12-c).

Dancing for one hour uses 250 calories. This varies according to the type of dance and the number of intervals between dances. The cha-cha, the quickstep and the Viennese waltz will burn more calories than the Bolero, depending of course on the way you dance!

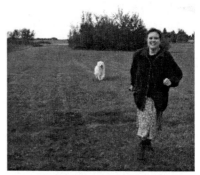

12-c Running the dog

Burning too many calories a week has been demonstrated to be hazardous for some people, and burning too few calories can also increase the risk of many diseases in others.

What is the ideal amount of exercise then for an average person?

According to many experts in the study of exercise, the ideal number of calories to burn in an average week to achieve close to a perfect balance of activity is 1500 to

2000. So, pick your favorite movement method, perform a simple calculation, and get active!

Now, the big problem arises when this patient, despite all these efforts, fails to lose excess body fat. It is at this point, and only when all other methods have failed, that the practitioner has to look at other treatments. These might include medications, or methods such as hypnosis. Medications, including both tablets and injections, are receiving much publicity, because now there is a lot more research being carried out into the causes and treatment of obesity. Consult your doctor for more information, because the possible side effects have to be considered before any of the available medications can be prescribed. The variety of tablets or capsules that can be prescribed can really help some patients a lot when other methods by themselves do not work.

There are about six medications that are prescribed, and all can work in selected patients. Some doctors are uncomfortable prescribing these types of medication, so they might prefer to refer you to a doctor who specializes in obesity.

In the process of weight/obesity control *be patient!* Do not expect large amounts of fat to disappear quickly. The small units that make up fat, which are called fat cells (adipocytes), are full of energy. When you are physically active, the fat cell is one of the last to give up its energy to this exercise! Your body uses amino acids (the building blocks for protein) and sugars (glucose) for the initial energy when exercising, leaving the fats in your body to be burned last!

Although the rate of weight loss varies, please do not expect to lose more than 5-10% of your weight in the first year. If you want to maintain this loss, allow *another* year of active treatment. It is a slow process to lose your excess weight, and you will have to keep to a correct eating/exercising routine forever. If proved to be safe, medication, or specialized counselling, might be needed regularly.

So, follow the meal plans from your doctor or dietician carefully and accurately and keep to your fitness system regularly.

Do You Worry? Are You Depressed or Anxious?

Emotions have a powerful effect, whether it be the rich and famous or the poverty-stricken; scholars or dunces, all are affected equally.

Depression can be a disease by itself, or it can be caused by other medical disorders, and it can be related, of course, to a bad life event, such as money problems, job loss or a death. Whatever the cause, finding a way to clear depression, along with other medical conditions that can be asso-

ciated with it, such as anxiety, obsessional-compulsive dis-
order/disease, alcoholism and a psychosis, is without any
doubt an essential goal.

Feeling depressed is a horrible experience, complications
are common, and the effect on the sufferer's own life, as
well as on those of their relatives and friends, is often extreme.

It must be stressed here that a cause should be looked for in
any of the symptoms of depression, or in its related symptoms such as panic, worry, fatigue and anger. As with any
unhealthy condition, an understanding of how a problem
started, that is, the medical history, is taken first. Then, a
total body examination and many other tests have to be
carried out.

A physical reason, as well as a social reason, could well be
the cause for the symptoms of worry, depression or anxiety. A serious example of a physical reason for a patient's
depression is a brain tumor! Hormonal imbalances, physical disabilities, severe persistent pain, and permanent organic disease are just a few additional identifiable reasons
for depression. In many people, a cause is not apparent.

Fortunately, for most people suffering from depression, a
serious underlying physical problem is not found. A cure

can be possible, and it might be as simple as treating an underactive thyroid gland.

It seems that many sufferers from depression have heard of various brain chemicals being the cause for their symptoms. In fact, it is these chemicals that are responsible for many types of so-called psychiatric disease. The chemicals that doctors refer to are called neurotransmitters, and simply put it is these nervous system substances that are out of balance and are the cause for the depression and the related disorders. Other mechanisms have been found to cause depression as well, mostly other chemicals from inside the brain cell being either too high or too low.

It is not known why these chemicals are thrown out of balance. In some diseases, such as Obsessional-Compulsive Disorder (OCD), there is evidence to suggest that cell damage is caused by bacterial toxins. Genetics is known to be a cause in some patients' depression, and in some others previous viruses might be the bullets that punctured the brain cell membranes.

Often a treatment in the form of a medication to correct that balance is necessary. Psychological methods, such as cognitive therapy, can help in anxiety, worry, fears and anger. As with many diseases, a single treatment will not work. With depression, it is necessary to help balance the chemicals back to normal. To achieve a correction of depression, another chemical has to be put into the body to rebalance the brain chemical. There are many prescribed chemicals (medicines) that can help, as well as a few herbal preparations. Prescription chemicals are more predictable in their effects, and have usually been more thoroughly tested for safety. Your own doctor should advise you on the correct choice if your diagnosis suggests that you need a medicine for depression.

To date, there is no simple test to assess which substances have to be balanced in the body. Such a test would be ideal, not only to diagnose depression but also to accurately treat the problem, with a guarantee that it will work well! It is reassuring to know that tests to detect these chemical imbalances are possible, but are not yet available for everyday use.

If you have heard of a Positron Emission Tomogram, or PET scan, as a test for depression, you are not imagining things. In the 1980s, tests were done in the eastern United States, and it was found that people with depression had a different scan compared with those who did not. Radioactive glucose was shown to be deficient in the front part of the brain in those patients suffering from depression. What is more, when these people were given anti-depressant medication, the brain glucose, as seen on the scanner, returned to normal. Because a PET scanner is extremely expensive to use, and because depression is so common, it might never be used to help diagnose depression.

Now, how is depression related to injuries?

It is observed, and clinical studies described in *Archives of Internal Medicine,* vol. 159, pp. 484-90, March 8, 1999, have confirmed, that depression has been found to be a cause for both *osteoporosis and fractures.* Therefore, depression can cause osteoporosis, which in turn can cause fractures, and depression can cause fractures independent of those fractures caused by osteoporosis.

To prevent both osteoporosis and fractures, along with all the other factors that cause osteoporosis or injuries (see the chapters on osteoporosis for those that we can influence), depression cannot be left untreated. Of course, the most common reason to treat depression is to relieve the sufferer of a terrible feeling, as well as to prevent the common complications of social damage (family breakup, job loss, loss of friends, etc), obesity in some, suicide risk, alcohol abuse, and many other health risks.

Chapter 13

More Important than Menopause — Perimenopause

Apart from birth or the onset of menstrual periods, most so-called stages of a woman's life are gradual, not sudden. Seemingly, perimenopause is one of the most gradual (there are, of course, always exceptions) natural changes I can think of that a woman has to go through. It is also one of the most important times to ensure that she has an understanding of what is needed to prevent the potential medical disorders that can occur at what *can be* a glorious time of life. Acquisition of important health information about hormone changes, along with the impact that they have on women, should be well understood, and nowadays it can be because of the tremendous amount of knowledge now available.

By the time of life that *the change* occurs, most women have acquired many life skills, have learned from their mistakes, and are necessarily wiser than they were. As always, combining knowledge and wisdom can certainly provide a powerful weapon to combat the medical disorders that could develop in the perimenopause.

Correct action taken during perimenopause is necessary to guard against preventable medical disorders that can occur in the menopause.

In other words, for most women, what you do in perimenopause will decide what will happen to you in menopause. A healthy, injury-free perimenopause opens the way for a healthy, injury-free menopause.

Obviously, before looking at the health issues of this time of life, it is necessary that we all talk the same language. Let us all agree on the meanings of words used so much by doctors, such as premenopause, perimenopause, natural menopause, postmenopause and the climacteric. The average woman or doctor will use terms such as menopause, change of life, the change, the turn of life, or, as alluded to above, *the age of wisdom.*

Premenopause

Premenopause describes the time from when your periods start to the menopause (see below for the meaning of menopause). Another way of describing this is that premenopause means those years of your life when you can have babies, or the reproductive time of life.

Perimenopause

This is the time between the onset of *any features* that suggest loss of the hormone estrogen, which usually means that the ovaries are not working normally, to the time when full menopause is obvious. A common question a doctor hears is this: "How old will I be when perimenopause starts?"

Perimenopause can start or precede menopause by about ten years, and it is not unusual to see women at age thirty-five starting with medical complaints that eventually turn out to be caused by a lack of estrogen.

Reduced ovarian hormone levels are suggested by any of the following three features:

1) There are symptomatic things that you might suffer, such as hot flushes or sudden sweating spells. Later in this chapter, a complete grouping of peri-menopausal/menopausal symptoms are provided in an A to Z list to help you to recognize or identify problems that you might be experiencing.

2) Other people — your spouse, a friend, your doctor or, of course, you — might see or recognize a change in your appearance or alterations in other aspects of your body. The change they see might be visible, or it could be a change in your emotions, in your drive, in your self- confidence or even in your personality.

3) Medical tests can *reveal* that your hormone levels are dropping, and these tests should include any

investigation for your medical complaints, such as one for anemia if you are bleeding excessively.

The single test most often done on the blood for menopause onset is called Follicle Stimulating Hormone (FSH), which is produced in a gland called the pituitary, a small, oval-shaped structure located near and connected to an area under the brain. This FSH stimulates the ovary to produce the hormone called estrogen in women. Your doctor can order this FSH blood level, and when the result is available you will note that the laboratory form will show a number followed by a symbol, usually "U/L." This abbreviated symbol refers to the number of units that there are of FSH in a liter of blood.

Your doctor will have to interpret the blood test result for you, but generally a higher FSH level on a blood test suggests a low availability of estrogen to the woman's body. For example, if the test shows a result such as 16 U/L, it is suggesting that the ovary is starting to *fail* (perimenopause), and when that number exceeds 40 U/L it is suggesting ovarian *shutdown* (menopause).

Thus, the beginning of perimenopause can be a feeling or symptom, a visible change, or a finding from a medical test.

Natural Menopause

After your periods have come to a complete stop, usually it means that your ovaries have stopped working altogether. If this occurs naturally, that is, not from the use of medicines, or from surgery or because of a disease, then after a year has passed the absence of a period means that you are in what is called natural menopause.

Postmenopause

Once you know that you have finished your periods, that is, one year has passed with no normal menstruation, it is from this time on that you are in what is called post-menopause.

The Climacteric

Usually, this term refers to the time in a woman's life after menopause, in other words, it has the same meaning as postmenopause. There are many experts though who maintain that the word climacteric means the time of life when the ovaries start to lose their effect (the same meaning as perimenopause).

The confusion over the meaning of the term the climacteric has led experts to decide to stop using the word; therefore, it is unlikely that you will see this word in modern magazines or books.

If you are at the perimenopause time of life, you might have few to no symptoms, or you might have one or more of a variety of quite different complaints. To simplify this variety of symptoms, the A to Z list below illustrates a large number of the problems that a woman could suffer from as a result of a drop in the estrogen levels in the body structures. *Remember this though — do not assume that a medical problem has only one cause!* Many of the listed medical problems that occur at the age of female hormone change, that is, thirty-five years and up, can have other causes. For example, back or heel pain can be caused by an estrogen lack, or it could be from totally unrelated conditions, such as arthritis, bone spurs, and many more disorders.

So, it is a combination of symptoms, proved to be not caused by any other disease, that can lead to the conclusion that perimenopause has started.

Check with your doctor to help verify whether or not your medical problems are hormone related. *It can actually be quite a relief* to find that a whole bunch of symptoms that you have been worrying about for months turn out to have been caused by perimenopause alone. For example, you have crawling feelings all over your face, you experience an irritable mood, and you are extremely tired all the time. After consulting the Internet, you are sure you have multiple sclerosis. A visit to the doctor, however, confirms that the symptoms you are experiencing are all due to perimenopause. What a relief!

An important point to remember about any unpleasant medical problem, if persistent, and even if *originally* diagnosed as perimenopausal, is that it needs to be examined again, repeatedly if necessary, to make sure that another medical problem is not *copying* the symptoms of perimenopause. For example, a mild, low back pain is at first found to be caused by a lack of female hormone estrogen. Treatment helps at first, but as time passes a vertebra or a disc slips, worsening instead of improving the back pain. Obviously, this continuing pain would be re-examined, an additional diagnosis would be made, and then obviously a suitable method of treatment would be recommended and followed.

Do Perimenopausal/Menopausal-associated Problems Need Treatment?

One of the most common questions asked about menopause and anything related to it is the one above. Sometimes just checking to make absolutely sure that a woman's medical problems are not the result of serious illness is enough to settle some of the fears that occur around this time of life. *Worry* can be part of estrogen lack, so talking to an expert who can check for disease, diagnose your symptoms, and thoroughly advise you is extremely important. This same, preferably medical, adviser can then, of course, discuss the question of need for treatment.

Whether a woman has symptoms or not, there has to be an agreement between the patient and health practitioner on the need to treat with a particular therapy. The need for treatment, in other words, is a joint decision that is often based on many factors.

Generally, there has to be a benefit of some kind for the patient when deciding on a therapy, whether of one or more varieties, and although this might sound like an obvious statement a medical adviser has to justify any treatment, especially if it has any type of risk.

So, to summarize, perimenopause/menopause can manifest itself in the three ways listed above, which again are feelings of body or mental changes (symptoms), visible changes in yourself (signs), or medical tests that show loss of female hormones.

Once you realize that perimenopause is happening, or that menopause has started, and you are feeling unwell from the lack of female hormones in any way, then some sort of medical help should be sought. As with any therapy, the symptoms or signs that interfere with your life are usually treated, as long as it is safe to do so!

Some of the unpleasant feelings that people can suffer have been mentioned briefly as the symptoms of perimenopause. For the sake of simplicity, as well as of reference, these hormone-related, sometimes unpleasant sensations can be put into an A to Z list. Check through this list for yourself or for a friend.

The A to Z List of Perimenopause Symptoms:

A: Anger; awaking with sore heels

B: Breast problems; bloating

C: Confusion; crying easily

D: Depression; dizzy spells

E: Easily upset

F: Fears

G: Gain in weight (obesity)

H: Hot flashes; headaches

I: Insomnia and strange dreams

J: Joint pains and muscle pain

K: Kyphosis (spine bending forward because of soft bone)

L: Lapses of memory

M: Menstrual irregularities

N: Nervousness

O: Osteoporosis

P: Prickly skin (crawly feelings in face); palpitations

Q: Questions about what is happening, and what to do about them

R: Rogue chin hairs

S: Sexual problems

T: Tiredness; thinning hair

U: Urgency of passing urine, and other bladder problems

V: Vaginal dryness/painful sexual intercourse

W: Worry; waking up early

X: X-rays show mid-back fractures (causing back pain)

Y: Yeast or other vaginal infections/allergies

Z: Zest for life drops off

It has now been decided that, after looking at a list of medical problems, after having had a thorough medical examination, and after assessing the blood tests, you are diagnosed with perimenopause. So, what is the next step? What you do at this point depends on how you feel, as well as on your personal preferences, that is, your life view in general, your religious beliefs, your health knowledge, etc.

The three menopause category situations that you could be part of are as follows:

1) You feel well, so you just simply continue to live in a healthy way, to eat good quality food, and to enjoy exercise in a way that helps all your body systems (for both, refer to Chapters 7 and 10, and Chapters 16 to 20). Regular medical examinations do help to detect hidden disease, as well as update you on important health facts.

2) If you have any of the perimenopausal symptoms in the A to Z list that are making your life difficult, then a remedy should be looked at. Please discuss your need for help with your health practitioner and see the suggestions listed below.

3) In this situation, you have symptoms, but do not wish to take any prescribed therapy, either from a doctor or from a non-physician source (for example, a health food store). This avoidance of therapy is, of course, all right, as long as you are not suffering from some of the more serious problems caused by estrogen imbalance, which would include long episodes of vaginal bleeding, serious infections, a fracture, or even deep depression. To avoid suffering, or even death,

these situations need medical help. If your problems prove not to be extreme, then the healthy living approach shown in the first category above would apply.

For each and every symptom in the A to Z list above, there is usually a remedy of some sort that can be recommended to give relief.

The next chapter looks at a selection of those upsetting problems that match the A to Z list, along with a variety of remedies that can help.

Preventing falling injuries, as is often mentioned, is the objective of every chapter. It will be noted that a lot of the information shown does not seem to be directly relevant to the topic of human injury; but, for completion of an extremely important subject, some other features of perimenopause are included that can be treated if the need arises.

Chapter 14

Remedy Guide for Perimenopause — The A to Z List

Upsetting changes in a woman's health at age thirty-five
and up are not always because of just a hormone
imbalance. Changes in the home and at work are possible
disturbers of health, as is the natural aging process, because
the longer that we are around or alive the greater the
chance of acquiring health problems. A natural change
that upsets many of us who are lucky enough to reach and
advance beyond middle age is the arrival of those visible
changes of approaching old age; it is amazing how many
people suffer psychological effects from this as they
advance in years. When among the middle-aged, younger
people seem to assume that these people, forty-five and up,
are content with their looks, as well as with the way they
feel at that time of life. In fact, deep down, some older
people can be extremely upset by their advanced age, and
depression and grumpiness can result.

Changes in the home include, of course, any children in
the family who are getting older, and all these can cause a
compound alteration in the interaction between a child
and a parent. A male partner can, of course, experience
health changes caused by a disease process, or by the
natural andropause. Friction created between two people in

the same home with health upsets is a setting for double trouble.

As you might gather from the above comments, correcting any medical problems that occur at the age of perimenopause is not as easy as taking female hormones.

The following list is a collection of medical complaints that I see regularly in my practice. It is by no means complete, but it does cover many poor-health issues that many women are likely to encounter.

A Remedy List for Many Perimenopausal Problems

Anger: This word means different things to different people. Whether it be mad at the world, upset over minor situations or experiencing emotional swings, this condition is not rare. Once a woman realizes that this is a problem, there are many kinds of help: specialized counseling, anger management classes, medications such as tryptophan (an important amino acid), various types of antidepressants, aerobic activities (including dancing — a message to all men!), correcting hormone imbalances and sleep disorders, avoiding alcohol, and practising relaxing sports such as yoga or tai chi. The list of possibilities is long, and can be used along with expert help. Incidentally, the risk of injuries is higher when a person is constantly upset.

Awaking with Sore Heels: This has a number of causes. If discomfort in the rear part of the foot is because of a hormone imbalance, treatment for this with a short course of estrogen replacement can be considered, assuming that other treatments have been tried and that there is no reason to avoid that type of therapy. Painful heels can both affect stability and contribute to the risk of a fall injury, so correcting footwear, using shoe inserts (orthotics), and applying medical treatments such as injections, as well as other remedies of the physical therapy type, can all be tried.

Breast Problems: Be on high alert for breast cancer with *careful* breast examinations. Beware of false-negative mammograms, because this test can miss seeing both small and large breast cancers! Painful, lumpy and swollen breasts are fairly common, but all these symptoms have to be assessed and treated by a physician.

There is no general therapy for breast disorders. Each woman's complaint has to be assessed and treated as a disease until it can be proved to be a benign condition, and only then can the disorder be managed.

Bloating: Intestinal gas (flatus) is a common cause for this complaint and, as with many other possible estrogen deficient symptoms, a medical examination, perhaps with tests, is a must. If natural gas is found to be the cause, there are some basic rules to be followed. Similarly, some not too serious colon disorders, such as diverticular disease, are associated with more than the usual bloating. Here are some general rules for those situations where no medical disorder has been found.

Check for the inability to digest *lactose* by trying to avoid milk or milk products, and use a lactase enzyme such as "Lactaid". This condition, well-known as lactose intolerance, does vary in incidence in different racial groups.

Fructose is added to pop or soft drinks, is found in fruits, as well as in other natural substances such as honey and jams. Try taking this away from your diet temporarily as a self-test, or get medical investigations to see if this is your bloating cause.

Sorbitol can be found in fruits, chewing gum, mints and other sweetened products. Avoiding this substance is worth the effort in an attempt to control annoying and unwanted flatus.

Lactose, fructose and sorbitol are all types of sugars, and eliminating these from your daily diet, as already mentioned, will give you a clue as to whether or not they are causing your gas. A test, called a hydrogen breath test, can also be carried out to help to diagnose the problem.

Almost any excessive amount of starch-type foods (which are complex sugars), can cause unwanted bowel gases. The starches that are not fully digested are attacked by bacteria, after this a type of fermentation takes place, which releases gases such as hydrogen, carbon dioxide and even methane into the intestine. Starches that do seem to be well absorbed, that is, leave little residue to be fermented, are rice and gluten-free products, such as breads and cakes that use gluten-free flour.

In the same way that bacteria digest leftover starches, excess proteins and certain vegetable or plant materials can also produce these distending gases from fermentation processes.

Swallowing air, sometimes caused by anxiety, or just as part of a habit such as chewing gum, can also cause bloating.

Irritable bowel syndrome, with or without constipation, is associated with bloating, but there is help for this with a variety of prescribed medicines. Often just controlling constipation is enough to help those many sufferers of being "full of wind."

Activated charcoal, which has been used for decades for unwanted gas, should also be tried, and over-the-counter products that contain digestive enzymes are useful for some people.

Certain exercises can help to stop the buildup of gas pressure. If you look at the *5x5 Mix* section, the rolling methods are excellent for dispersing the gas bubbles in your intestine and thereby allowing release.

Confusion: This is an important problem to have checked medically. If it is caused by a lack of estrogen, and if there is no reason to avoid this hormone, then a trial of this treatment could be helpful (see section on hormone remedies below).

Regular physical activity and relaxation methods, including yoga and tai chi, can help to improve concentration abilities a lot, thus reducing confusional states.

A common complaint that I see as a doctor is the patient who is upset by the loss of the ability to make decisions easily. These patients minds are jumbled by too many thoughts, so that they become confused as to how to progress from hour to hour.

Relaxation methods can help this, as can the temporary use of a calming agent, such as tryptophan or a short-acting sedative. A good psychologist can help to direct you, and can teach you ways to focus on the right thing at the right time by using various types of treatment, including cognitive therapy.

Crying Easily: Depression can cause this problem, but it is not, of course, a condition that is seen only in menopause. More details on the serious and common medical disorder of depression can be read in Chapter 12, as well as in the next description.

Depression: Depression is a common but critically important disorder at *all* ages. A variety of other diseases can cause depression, including serious disorders such as brain tumors. If you suffer from this condition, you should get a thorough medical examination, and then appropriate therapy can be offered. With correct treatment, you should feel well; in fact, you should be able to be your normal self again. Along with counseling, medication and aerobic-type exercise, you should not only feel well but also lessen your risk of falling and fracturing bones.

Dizzy Spells: Obviously, this is of great importance, not only as an upsetting feeling but also as a risk for falling. Tests, with a thorough medical checkup, are necessary to unravel the cause for this serious symptom. If the problem is because of a hormone deficiency (estrogen/progesterone), the practising of medically advised exercises can help, along with the benefits to be gained from the rotational types of activities seen in the *5x5 Mix* (see Chapters 16 to 20).

Easily Upset: Refer to the "Anger" section above for this problem.

Fears: A psychologist who specializes in this group of disorders can help, using techniques such as cognitive therapy or hypnosis. In some people, estrogen-type compounds (gels, patches, tablets and injections) can help, at least until other treatments start to work. A physician would help with this decision.

Gain in Weight (Obesity): This is a popular topic because it is an extremely common misery for so many women. There is a tendency to gain excess fat with advancing years: the average person, male or female, gains at least a quarter of a pound (eighth of a kilogram) a year. So, it is not surprising that, by the "age of wisdom," this collection of extra insulation is more noticeable.

For some people, getting their waist measurements back to normal values is relatively easy; for others, however, it seems to be impossible. True obesity, thought of by some scientists as a disease, that is, appetite and the chemicals that *make* fat in our bodies are affected by our genes, should be *medically* assessed at first by your physician. A medical interview, an examination and tests might be necessary. Then, if no other medical condition is found, a weight/fat reduction system can be planned, perhaps with help from various health experts. This plan could include regular visits to a medical doctor, a correct long-term nutrition regimen monitored by a dietitian, and adequate exercise, counseling and, sometimes, prescribed medication.

Be prepared to continue your excess body weight control for many years, and please do not expect to lose large amounts of fat quickly (see Chapter 12 for more information).

Hot Flashes: Although these sudden episodes of often extreme warmth, felt and seen in the face, as well as in other areas of the body, are tolerated by some women, they are unbearable to others. Sudden flushing, noticeable to other people as a red flare in the face, sometimes with instantaneous flooding of the skin with sweat, is a miserable experience.

Sufferers demand help! Control of these symptoms is possible with a variety of therapies, assuming that these hot spells are of the menopausal type.

Non-hormonal — Prescription type: Clonidine, for example, Dixarit, Bellergal and Venlafaxine (Effexor, also an anti-depressant)

Non-hormonal — Non-prescription type: The use of Black Cohosh and Dong Quai should be discussed with your doctor, especially if you plan on taking it long term.

Hormonal — Prescription type: Estrogens of many types. These compounds, in certain women, can be safe. Generally, the safest estrogen medications are the type that are absorbed through the skin, such as gels and patches. As most women know, side effects are possible from using replacement estrogen, but they can be minimized by considering each patient's risks separately.

Measures such as avoiding smoking, eating correctly, exercising, carrying out regular breast self-examination, minimizing alcohol intake, and taking progesterone if you have a uterus all help to reduce some of the complications that can occur with female hormones. It is known that the individual factors that can aggravate adverse effects of estrogen are also in themselves potentially dangerous. Alcohol and lack of exercise are both thought to increase the risks of developing breast cancer more than that of taking estrogen.

Anyone who has suffered the heat and flash flooding of estrogen deficiency, but who also has total control of it with hormone therapy, will tell you that they will not stop the treatment because their quality of life at the present time is more important than caring about any *possible* future risks.

Many of the serious possible side effects of estrogen replacement therapy tend to occur after four to five years of use.

Hormonal — Non-prescription type: There are various brands available. Most are prepared from yams, soybeans or red clover. Because these over-the-counter menopausal aids do consist of estrogen, side effects are to be considered in the same way as any other female hormone product.

When considering research or studies that involve hormones, as well as the advice that they provide, and especially when the information has been interpreted by the media, look to your own physician for help and guidance. In 2002, the Women's Health Initiative (WHI) study caused many women to worry excessively, mostly because of the way that the media had presented the results. So, please discuss studies such as the WHI one with your own doctor.

Headaches: Many headaches are caused by more than one factor at the same time, and they are then called *mixed headaches.* When considering how to treat a headache, a doctor has to determine *all* the possible causes.

Many estrogen deficiency headaches are a mixture of head muscles contracting and blood vessels swelling.

Treatments can involve the use of massage therapy, acupuncture, muscle relaxants, antimigraine medicines of various types, estrogen preparations, pain control therapies, relaxation methods, as well as what are called biofeedback methods. In addition, regular physical activity can also help to prevent some types of headache.

Insomnia and Strange Dreams: Sleep problems can be caused by other perimenopausal upsets or by a single condition. If any doubt exists as to the cause for the insomnia, ideally a sleep study should be carried out.

For help with this draining situation, get a list of sleep hygiene rules. This list includes suggestions such as avoiding caffeine or activities that stimulate the brain or body at sleep time, using the bedroom for relaxing or sleeping only, along with similar ideas that help to rid you of slumber destroyers. Aids that help to promote good quality sleep have not changed much over the years. Hypnosis, meditation systems, sleep potions (valerian root and diphenhydramine), pharmaceutical products, estrogen therapy, and many other homespun ideas, such as reading a story designed to induce sleep, can all help insomnia in certain individuals who need treatment. If despite sleeping a person still remains unrefreshed, a medical consultation should be sought. Medical disorders such as depression or sleep apnea could be issues that need special help. As mentioned, a variety of sleep disorders that need special treatment might be discovered with a sleep analysis, which can be ordered with the help of your doctor and by referral to a sleep disorder specialist.

Fatigue from insomnia is a recipe for physical injuries, so get help!

Incidentally, unusual dreams can be settled with many of the above remedies as well, but according to some authors such dreams should be recorded, and might well turn into a best-selling novel!

Joint Pains and Muscle Pains: Symptoms of this type, of course, need an accurate diagnosis. If these pains are because of menopause, various methods are known to help. Raising the body's sex hormones to their normal levels can help, but if these hormones cannot be used there are other alternatives: massage treatments, vibration therapy, muscle strengthening exercises (see exercise

Chapters 17 to 20), herbal or prescribed anti-inflammatory substances, acupuncture, injection therapies (often given at pain clinics), special creams, liquids and gels that can be self-applied, and mechanical aids and braces that temporarily support joints to help in activities.

Please see your health practitioner for more ideas, and to help *to diagnose* the possible causes as well.

Kyphosis (Spine Bending Forward Usually Because of Soft Bone): This forward curvature of the spine is disfiguring, uncomfortable, reduces the quality of life, throws off the balance, and can affect internal organ functioning. Prevention is, as usual, the best approach to this life-threatening condition. Attention to osteoporosis, posture, abdominal muscle strength, pain control and diet are all important factors in the preventive ideas to avoid kyphosis (see osteoporosis, Chapters 6 and 7).

Lapses of Memory: Revealing the reasons for this scary disorder is most important. Menopausal causes for amnesia can be helped with female hormone replacement (of the many types, and with the usual precautions), as can maintaining high fitness levels and good nutrition (fish, nuts, pasta, and extra vitamins such as B_{12} and B_6). Memory challenging exercises can all help as well. If there is doubt, however, as to the cause for the amnesia episodes, specialized memory clinics do exist for more advanced assessment and help. Ginkgo biloba and ginseng are claimed to help some people, but if long-term treatment is planned the side effects should be considered under the care of an expert in the use of herbal remedies.

Menstrual Irregularities: Serious diseases can be the culprit here, so it is necessary to have a medical checkup for this common upset, at any age from the beginning of menstruation (menarche) to the arrival of menopause.

When the cause for any abnormal menstrual bleeding is proved to be because of hormone imbalance, the situation can be settled in a few ways: by balanced female hormone replacement (estrogen with progesterone); by short-term use of the contraceptive pill; by a curettage (scraping) of the uterine lining, otherwise called a D&C; and sometimes by achieving control of a menstrual cycle using an arthritis medicine called Anaprox DS. With many experiences, I have found that the copy, or generic, version of this drug does not work to control heavy menstruation or painful periods. So, if you try this temporary aid, insist on the correct brand name. Those of you that are allergic to aspirin, have blood disorders, stomach ulcers or similar should avoid this type of medication. (This statement is based on my personal experience and is an opinion that may not be felt by other medical doctors. Consult your own physician for advice on this matter.)

There are permanent treatments for the above problems, but see your doctor for up-to-date methods, and do not forget that heavy bleeding causes loss of iron from your body, which can lead to anemia.

Nervousness: Lack of confidence, anxiety and worry can all be included here.

Reassurance, relaxation methods and various medications (including estrogen if safe), all mentioned above, can be beneficial; moreover an understanding and knowledgeable family, as well as friends and associates, that is, help from every direction possible, can go a long way to make this symptom tolerable.

Osteoporosis: When I find this disease process in a person, I compare it with a situation where the bones are aging or dying before the rest of the body. The chapter on osteoporosis has a complete description of this dangerous and common disease.

Palpitations: If you have the feeling that your heart is beating extra hard or extra fast, you are experiencing palpitations. These heart sensations have to be listened to by a doctor, and if necessary tests such as electrocardiograms are ordered. If these, often worrisome, chest sensations are caused by a lack of female hormone, there are a number of choices for controlling this type of palpitation. Reassurance sometimes is enough; just knowing that you are not about to have a heart attack can often reduce fear, thus slowing the heart speed. Taking magnesium tablets or liquid can control a speeding heart as well, as can injections of vitamin B_{12} in certain patients.

More often than not, a low dose of estrogen will fully control this upsetting feeling. Occasionally, a heart medicine can be given that blocks receptors to the heart, thus settling the speed, and in turn reduces the uncomfortable sensation. Avoidance of all stimulants, such as sources of caffeine, alcohol, nose decongestants and nicotine, as well as excitement or fatigue, can help to successfully clear palpitations (see illustration 14-a).

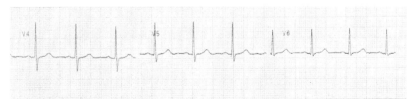

14-a ECG tracing — As part of an assessment of palpitations, an ECG is necessary to help exclude a heart disorder. This is a reminder that heart disease is still a serious and common problem for women.

Prickly Skin: Described in the previous chapter, this feeling is not usually severe; it is more of a curiosity for the woman who feels as if there are ants crawling on her face.

Questions about Menopause: There are always more questions on this topic than answers. I cannot answer all the questions on the subject of menopause, and certainly not in just one chapter. Medical research will continue to provide answers to some of the menopause puzzles that we still have to solve.

In the meantime, keep your ears and eyes open, make use of old and new information that benefits your mind and body, and thereby extend your healthy years!

Rogue Chin Hairs: Most women dislike spiky chin or other facial hairs. Have your doctor check for the causes of unwanted facial hair, and then look at various treatments that are available, such as electrolysis and prescription medicine (Aldactone occasionally helps), or just pluck the hairs out regularly.

Sexual Problems: See Chapter 15, entitled Perimenopausal Sex — 'In a Nutshell.'

Tiredness: Please see the section on fatigue in Chapter 12.

Thinning Hair: Scalp and body hair thinning has a number of causes. Female hormone *imbalance* is often a cause for thinning scalp hair, and correcting this imbalance can help in some women. A medical checkup is necessary to ensure that no scalp disease or other general medical disorder is causing the hair to thin, which can often include even the eyebrows. Thyroid disease should also be considered in the list of causes.

There are a few scalp therapies available that could help, such as Minoxidil, along with prescriptions. In addition, hair implants can be tried if all other therapies fail. See your physician for help or a referral to a specialist, but remember that, in some women, and with the passage of time alone, hair loss will often regrow!

Urinary Problems: Urinary leakage caused by weak pelvic muscles and thin skin and membranes in the pelvic region, along with other upsets, such as pelvic heaviness (a prolapse of the vagina is one cause), can all be helped. The pelvic muscles should be made stronger with any method that is available to you, and could include special vaginal weights, specialized physiotherapy, and Kegel-type exercises. Differently shaped pessaries for the vagina and special valves for the urethra can all be tried before medication or surgery is considered for a leaky bladder.

Medical remedies include female hormone replacement (in the form of creams, tablets, patches or injections), and drugs that help the bladder to be less irritable or overactive. Bladder disease, including all symptoms, should be investigated medically before any surgical treatment is started.

Vaginal Dryness/Painful Sexual Intercourse: This is a common concern around the time of menopause.

As long as there are no medical reasons to avoid it, estrogen cream, instilled every four days, can be extremely helpful for vaginal dryness or itching.

Around menopause, the cells of the vaginal skin are reduced in number and change to a thinner shape. Along with cell change, the blood flow in the vaginal wall is reduced. Estrogen cream inserted into the vagina will increase the layers of cells and improve the blood flow, thereby improving the general health of the vagina. Itching and dryness should clear, as well vaginal lubrication with sexual activity will improve, as often will sexual desire. Generally, it is found that, just with the use of the vagina in sexual activity, natural lubrication and engorgement of the erectile tissue of the vulva are improved.

Worry: This is discussed in the "Nervousness" and "Depression" sections.

Waking up Early: Early morning awaking can be caused by depression. Using the approach listed in the "Insomnia" and "Depression" sections is necessary.

Hormone replacement therapy (estrogen) can help, as well as the medications Desyrel (Trazodone), occasionally Effexor (Venlafaxine, initially this can sometimes worsen a sleep disorder), or similar choices, but these, of course, have to be prescribed.

X-rays: If done to find the cause for back pain, a side view x-ray of the spine could reveal a collapse of a vertebra (a block of the spine being crushed because of thinning of the bony structure, namely osteoporosis).

Bone densitometry is a test that uses weak x-rays to assess the skeleton for signs of osteopenia or osteoporosis.

Yeast Infections: Vaginal yeast infections can be a nuisance at any age. Remedies include antiyeast vaginal creams or vaginal tablets called pessary medications, capsules taken by mouth that need a prescription, and vaginal paintings with gentian violet, a therapy that can be provided by a medical doctor.
Immunotherapy injections to Candida albicans can help many women with recurrent yeast vaginitis, but allergy tests are needed to obtain this treatment, and these should

be carried out by a doctor who is knowledgable in this type of remedy.

As usual, if vaginal irritation persists despite therapy, a medical examination is necessary.

Zest for Life Reduced: Many of the problems described above that are caused by a lack of estrogen do not always occur. There are plenty of women who sail through perimenopause and menopause feeling and staying healthy. If one or more of the above situations does occur, however, it is likely that it is going to affect the life quality of the sufferers.

Ideally, then, it is important for *every woman to have a deep understanding of the processes that concern the "change of life,"* so that a suitable remedy can be used when necessary, thereby directing women back onto a course of *health* and *happiness.*

Chapter 15

Perimenopausal Sex — 'In a Nutshell'

Before looking at some ideas on how to help many of the possible undesirable effects of female hormone imbalance, I would like to tell you a story about risky sex.

My first experience in helping to treat a sexual problem was when I was a medical student in England. To cut a long story short, a young couple attended our infertility clinic, but the tests did not reveal a cause for the woman's inability to get pregnant.

It was another not-so-shy student who solved the young couple's 'infertility' problem with one simple question. He simply asked them *how* they performed their sexual act! Their answer was not only embarrassing for the young couple but also caused some blushing faces in those specialists who, with all their experience, should have asked the same basic question of the "need-to-be parents," *before* doing all the medical tests.

This was their simple, yet innocent, answer to the medical student's basic question. The man, as ignorant about sex as his wife, was attempting to push his penis and scrotum into her belly button (navel)!

Of course, this story is not directly related to injuries or to perimenopause, but it certainly could result in a serious injury if people were to attempt the above couple's method of copulation in a passionate way. After this revelation, this young couple did get good advice, and they did eventually achieve a pregnancy.

Sexual Concerns

As human beings living in an imperfect world, we do suffer problems such as illnesses, injuries, emotional stress — you get the idea. Whether you have a problem or you are merely aware of problems through friends or the media, you must know that sexually related problems do exist, and what is more these disorders are not rare!

Some individuals and couples avoid sexual activity totally on purpose! They practise sexual abstinence or celibacy, just like monks and nuns in certain religious orders. Some couples and single people are not the slightest bit interested in sexuality at all, and are quite content with their situations.

Sexual concerns in individuals or couples are extremely varied; moreover, the sufferers are not always discovered, that is, they do not always share their problems with either health professionals or friends.

A not uncommon finding is a woman who claims that sexual topics are overrated one moment only to need sex voraciously in her life the next. This type of *normal* behavior is likely due to a combination of hormonal swings, along with environmental effects. Many women are highly sexual: some all the time, and others only if the right atmosphere or conditions are present for the sexuality to be expressed or released.

What Then Is a "Sexual Concern"?

This topic is so extensive that the scope has to be limited to long-term relationships between a man and a woman. There are many subjects of great importance, such as sexual deviations and problems within homosexual relationships. Readers seeking information on these topics, and sexually related diseases, should seek advice from their library, from a specialist in this area, or from a website with an author who is qualified to give out such information.

Our situation is a couple where either the woman or the man has a concern of any kind with their sexual life. Their concerns might be a long-term problem or a developing problem. They might have always had an unsatisfactory situation, or it could be a change from a highly sexual life to a life with a significantly reduced to a no-love-life existence.

Sexuality conjures up different thoughts in different people. Most people would think that it refers to the act of sexual intercourse (coitus), and some would think of it as looking or feeling sexy. The average adult, without a dictionary, would probably describe this term in a different way again to another adult, because the word sexuality means different things to different people.

Here are some meanings of sexuality:

Looking/feeling attractive

A woman and man having sexual intercourse

Moving (walking or dancing) in a sexy way

Having thoughts about sex

Cuddling, petting and kissing without genital involvement

Masturbation

Love or equivalent meanings

Smelling attractive

Pleasing the opposite sex in any way (gifts, flowers, etc)

Giving or receiving sexual pleasure in multiple ways (oral, anal, etc)

The list does not stop here, but we do have to proceed with our discussion.

Referring to the above list, we can now say that a sexual concern or problem exists if either a woman or her partner has a change for the worse in any of the above situations or in the equivalent ideas of what sex means to that couple. For practical purposes, the common sexual concerns will be looked at in this issue, especially in women age thirty-five years and up.

A List of Some of the Top Sexual Concerns

Loss of sexual feelings and thoughts

A dry vagina

Painful intercourse

Too tired to have sex/depressed

Feeling too fat or unattractive

Genital sensation lost/numb clitoris

Bad vaginal odors

Difficulty with sexual positions because of pain in the joints or abdomen

Hot sweats interfering with intimacy

Lack of sexuality in the partner (no romance, poor erections, etc)

Inability to have an orgasm, which might have always been a problem or might be a new worry

Vaginal bleeding

A genuine concern occasionally seen in a doctor's clinic is that of a woman who is upset over her inability to be satisfied sexually with just one orgasm! She might need to repeat that sexual experience, over and over again, as frequently as every five or ten minutes. This situation, of course, is a problem for her partner as well. There are various causes for this type of 'complaint.' Often the cause might be a yeast infection or other genital irritation, or it could be a hormone imbalance (there are various types), or it could even be a psychological problem. This, as with many of the above concerns, should be shared with your physician and checked for a medical cause.

Health problems such as depression or anxiety can be a cause or a result of reduced sexual ability. All the above complaints can be caused by a lack of female hormones, or at least an imbalance of those hormones. Hormonal change, however, is not the cause for all loss of or variation in sexual functioning. So, before deciding how best to correct or improve a changed sex life, other causes should be looked at first.

This Diagram Shows Groups of Factors that Affect

Sexual Appetite or Enjoyment

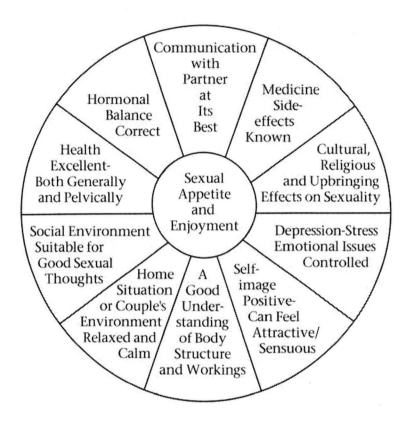

Although the above diagram of causes appears complete, there are many other possible causes for change in a person's sexual feelings. Every couple or individual who suffers a problem in any health area will have a unique situation that needs help, and so they will have to have unique therapy. The following notes can be used as a starting point or guide to help advise you about symptoms of possible perimenopause, with or without sexual concerns. In some areas, it might offer a complete remedy for some of the upsets listed that can cause long-term health issues.

Generally, a woman in a good or happy relationship is easier to help with any sexual problem than one in an unsettled marriage or equivalent partnership. I rarely think of a sexual concern as belonging to a woman or to a man, because it is a *shared* problem.

To be able to treat or help a woman with concerns with her love life, it is helpful to describe or group these concerns. Is the problem severe or is it mild? Are there any obvious factors that affect or are related to this loss of sexuality? Is this problem a single concern or a whole list of worries?

The easy reference chart shown below is a guide only, but it has been designed to help anyone with a sex-related worry to possibly find a solution to that concern.

It is a curious fact, but in health matters generally people can look the same and have the same type of blood, yet their bodies can behave quite differently under the same conditions. Whether it is a reaction to a medication or behavior under different hormonal conditions, opposite effects can be seen. An appetite suppressant can work well in one person, but in another it can actually stimulate the appetite. Sexual appetite can behave the same way. It can be absent for days to years, only to return suddenly to normal, and sometimes for no obvious reason.

Knowing that sex problems can be temporary, along with acknowledging that most of them have a cause, medical help is always possible.

The "nutshell" diagrams shown here are a guide only for the concerned person to follow.

A healthy sexual existence should be considered as part of the normal sphere of life. (This sphere, an efficient shape in nature, is perfect when life is perfect, and it should expand smoothly with pleasant life experiences.)

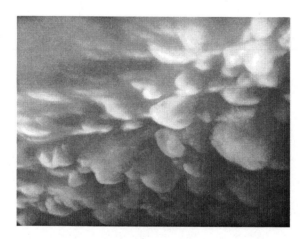

The Top Nutshell

	The Worry	The Cause	The Remedy
The	Pain with any portion of the sexual act	Disease of any part of the genitals. Psychological causes possible	Treat the disease. Sexual counseling needed and help with psychological problems
	Vaginal dryness	Lack of estrogen is the most common cause	Estrogen cream for the genital area can help. Non-hormone moisturizers can be used. Sex activity can be lubricating
Sexual	Lack of sensation of the genital parts — a numb clitoris	Sex hormone imbalance is the likely cause. Nervous system diseases rarely are a cause	Testosterone and estrogen can help. Lubricants, clitoral vacuum devices, and Viagra can be used
	Desire for sex low or absent	Sex hormone imbalance, plus all the above factors	Any of the above, along with Desyrel or Wellbutrin, can help
Act	Genital parts, vulva seem shrunken	Lack of estrogen is the most common cause	Estrogen cream and transdermal estrogen. Lubrication with sexual activity helps
	Poor orgasm or no orgasm	Various causes possible. Often more than one cause is the reason. Psychological and hormone imbalance or disease possible	Sex education of the partners is needed. All aspects of sexual concerns have to be cared for (all the above apply), including masturbation ideas

Non-sex Act Concerns:	The Worry	The Cause	The Treatment
Communication/ Romance Issues	No sharing in activities, lack of caring, no romance. Issues not discussed	Upbringing, cultural issues, education, and life events	Counseling and education needed. Helpers' need to know cultures and religions of the various types
Direct Sex Act Concerns:			
Reduced Sexual Abilities Caused by: 1) Problems Mostly Psychological	Concerns about appearance with aging, body fat, shape. Anger, depression, anxiety, OCD	Needs a medical assessment	Counseling of both partners. Help with self-esteem. Drugs used for depression should be of the type that stimulate sexual desire
2) Problems Mostly of the Body Workings	Fatigue, unwell, pain of any type. Stiff hips, knees or other joints. Vaginal bleeding or discharge. Breathing or heart problems	Needs a medical assessment	A diagnosis has to be made, then the condition/illness treated with the sex issues considered in the treatment plan

The Bottom Nutshell

Just as good, quality food, correct exercise, education, and perfect physical and mental health are necessary to help us to feel well, sexuality is needed in many people to embellish their existence. Sex, no matter how one defines it, has many benefits, including its ability, when satisfactory, to aid in the completeness of a relationship between two people.

Further to the benefits of sexuality, medical studies have noted that health in various areas does improve with sexual activity. Improved vaginal skin lubrication and better blood flow in the erectile tissue of both women and men have been found. This improved blood flow delivers more oxygen to the genital area, producing healthier 'flesh'. There are also theories that suggest that a sexual act that culminates with an orgasm does help to reduce 'congestion' in the pelvic organs and veins; moreover, patients do indeed claim a relief in pressure sensations in the pelvis after satisfactory sexual acts.

Reduced chances of a heart attack have also been noted in some studies when a couple engage in sexual activity at least twice a week.

In men, according to some scientists, more ejaculations means less prostate cancer and perhaps a reduced risk of heart attacks!

Orgasms have been shown to stop any pain temporarily, although I cannot imagine anyone wanting sex when they are in pain (see orgasmic pain below). One often hears of the headache excuse for avoiding sex, but there are situations where some headaches actually clear with a pleasing episode of lovemaking.

A common benefit claimed of any kind of sex is that it helps to induce a state of deep relaxation and helps, at least temporarily, to alleviate depression. Another theory suggests that it is the chemicals in seminal fluid that lift one's spirits.

Sex is not the answer to everything, but it has a definite and beneficial place in life beyond that of reproducing.

The medical phenomenon of orgasmic pain in women is mentioned here to clarify that all orgasms are not always wonderful but can on rare occasions be quite unpleasant. There are situations where an orgasm can increase pressure in an area such as the head, making pressure-type headaches worse, or can increase spasms in tight muscles such as those in the back (in a back strain). These types of pain, when experienced with an orgasm, are pre-existing problems, and have not been directly caused by the orgasm; they are just aggravated by the excitement: blood pressure rising, adrenaline effects, and the tightening of muscles generally.

Orgasmic pain is pelvic discomfort where there was no previous problem. It is pain that is experienced during an orgasm, starting as the orgasm begins, and disappearing when the orgasm finishes. Like many sexual complaints, orgasmic pain has more than one cause. Frequently, there is an underlying emotional upset that acts as a factor for this uncommon pain, but some diseases of the pelvis can also be the culprit or cause. If there is a disease causing the orgasmic pain, obviously it must be treated, not only because of the potential health hazard of a pelvic disorder but also because it can turn off all interest in sexual activity.

A medical examination, along with at least an ultrasound of the pelvis, is essential when looking for a cause for pain of any type in the pelvic area. Some of the causes for orgasmic pain can include unhappy partner relationships, which might involve feelings of guilt, or other reasons why romance is lacking; tumor-type growths that press into the womb (uterus) or the muscles of the pelvic floor; and muscle strains that can occur in the muscles of the pelvic floor, in which case pain will only occur when these muscles contract, as in an orgasm. This condition should settle by purposely avoiding sexual activity for a while, after all treatments are complete. The information on this condition is based upon my own clinical experience, and to my knowledge there are no medical studies on this topic.

The orgasmic pain that is described here should not be confused with painful sexual intercourse, which is a totally different condition. A doctor has to diagnose the disease conditions that are possibly causing orgasmic pain. But remember, this is a rare condition.

Two Words to All Men: Communication and Romance

Do not forget these two words!

Talk in a gentle tone to your wife or your lover, whether it be good times or bad times.

Understand what medical problems women suffer from. Talk to her, and read with her about menopause. Tell her about *your* concerns in life. *Romance* means so much to most women, even when in a bad mood.

Here are some ideas to help with the romance in a relationship:

Give flowers with colors that your partner likes.

A woman's sense of smell is a strong feature in sex, whether it be flowers, the natural oils, sweat odors, including pheromones, or a scent that your partner likes. Enlist the aid of this sense often.

Take her dancing. If you cannot dance, learn by going for lessons together. Learn the *dance of love* — the rumba, and *dance sensually* — with the Argentine tango!

Go to the gym, or to almost any sports activity together.

Go for nice long walks in both sunshine and rain.

Make some tasty meals. If you cannot cook, go to classes.

Go out for meals to a good restaurant (but do not get drunk!).

Help by doing your share of the housework.

Shop for essential items together.

A relaxed woman can be extremely sexual, so slow down, and play some soft music.

If your lover has a problem in any sexual way, learn to understand what that problem is, what the possible causes are, and make sure that you show *patience* and understanding. It will benefit you and your female partner, because improvement in her sexual functioning *will* occur with the correct approach.

Men think of sex often (for a biological reason); women can think of sex often if they have the right atmosphere!

In other words, spend time together, and make the effort to share everything. A dynamite combination in a male/female relationship is the combination of love and all its meanings with healthy sex and all its meanings!

Chapter 16

A Beginner's Guide to the *5x5 Mix* Injury Prevention Activity System — Section One — The Warm-ups

Introduction to the Home Version

There is a missing element in the world of women's health care, and that is the omission of a serious approach that helps women to prevent body damage from physical injuries.

One has only to visit a few health clubs to see that there are lots of women exercising in many activity skills, such as yoga, Pilates, tai chi, aerobics and similar sports. The many sports activities that are available do provide excellent opportunities for women to stay fit and strong, to shed excess weight, and to maintain health in many ways.

Why do women attend, or not attend, regular fitness centers?

Many reasons exist for regularly attending physical fitness centers, including among others the drive to stay slim, to keep up fitness so as to avoid premature death, to feel well, and to use exercise as a hobby. For the many women who attend the fitness facilities regularly, there are just as many who do not seek fitness any-where, at a gym or at home. There are lists of reasons why scores of us are unfit: fatigue, disabilities, pain, fi-nances, and plain embarrassment about one's looks are just a few of the known excuses that prevent us from seeking out a fitness system and keep us in a downward spiral of poor health.

To help to supply the important aspects of women's health that are missing, the *5x5 Mix* system has been developed, not only to provide a complete fitness sys-tem that includes warm-ups, stretches, balance and strength training but also the gym or home level of training in Ground Reflex and Landing Skills (GRALS). The reflexes that can be developed from this system, once attained, can last for many years, perhaps forever!

In this and the next four chapters, only basic elements are shown. This version being the gym or home level of the *5x5 Mix*. Advanced reflex skills, as discussed in the individual chapters, include training outdoors, on hills, on ice, in the dark, and in environments with unex-pected objects that have to be avoided. These, along with the more acrobatic-type skills, are not described or demonstrated because they are too complex to learn — except, of course, for experts in the basic *5x5 Mix* sys-tem.

The following home version of the *5x5 Mix* is adequate to give fall injury prevention skills to those practising it, as well, their fitness level will improve. As always, repeat the reflex skills as shown as often as possible, and try to perfect them, because practice makes perfect, and then you can be armed with a system that will provide you with lasting abilities in the common world of this serious disease — fall injuries.

Music is of great help in developing a variety of rhythms with all the exercise groups described in these activity chapters. Suggested tunes should obviously suit each person's taste, but the tempos should be slow to moderate. The kinds of beat could follow the pattern of dance sounds: a 4/4 beat (swing, foxtrot, quickstep, and many pop tunes), and occasionally samba music helps you to keep moving (repeat the count "one-a-two"), or even a waltz (3/4 beat) is pleasant to work out to.

Part One — The Pro-Perfs (Warm-up Activity Guide)

First, the word "Pro-Perfs" should be defined: "Pro" refers to activities that stimulate the *pro*prioceptors, and "Perfs" are movements that improve blood flow through the muscles, therefore encouraging *perf*usion.

This group of movements helps to wake up the nerve endings (proprioceptors, the specialized nerve endings that make you aware of the positions of your body parts even with your eyes closed) and to open up the blood vessels in the muscles and skin, preparing your body for more dynamic activity. The heat generated by this group of movements helps tendons to stretch more easily, so that you are ready for the muscle toning and strengthening part of the *5x5 Mix.*

As in any physical activity, these warm-ups are necessary to avoid exercise-related strain injuries.

Air Grabs In the standing position, the feet should be shoulder width apart.

16-a Air grabs — hands open/relaxed

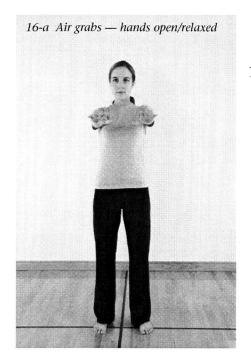

1) The arms outstretched, all fingers open, your fingers and shoulders should be relaxed (see photograph 16-a).

16-b Air grabs — tight fist

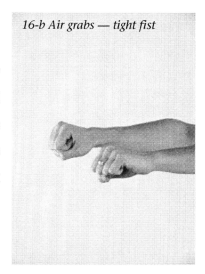

2) Close your fingers fairly tightly, forming a fist. Hold this fist position for two seconds, then straighten the fingers again. Repeat eight times (see photograph 16-b).

Pummeling Keep to the same position as Air Grabs.

1) Lightly slap the sides of the cheeks with the palms of your hands simultaneously, up to ten times (see photographs 16-c and 16-d).

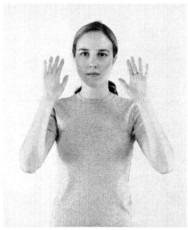

16-c Pummeling and the hand position to slap cheeks

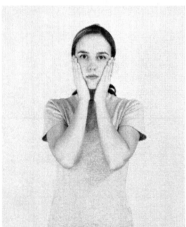

16-d Pummeling and the cheek slap

2) With a firm fist, you have to lightly pound simultaneously the left and right sides of your body.

Start by pounding the back of your left hand with your right fist, then continue along the side of your forearm, all the way up to the shoulder with that same right fist.

The tops of the shoulders can only be pummeled separately. The other hand (in the open palm position) can pound the opposite side of the chest simultaneously (the arms are crossed, one over the other). Pound each site five times: five times on the right shoulder with the left fist; five times on the left shoulder with the right fist. When pounding the back area, be careful that the impact falls close to the spine or over the low back, avoiding the kidney region (see photographs 16-e and 16-f).

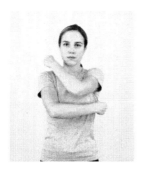

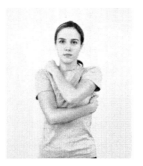

16-e Pummeling — pounding the right shoulder with the left fist and slapping the left chest with the right palm — before contact

16-f Pummeling, as in photograph 16-e, with contact

With a fist, lightly pound the lower back, the inner thighs, the outer thighs, and the sides of the lower legs, with all areas being pummeled about ten times (the right hand pounds the right side and the left hand pummels the left side of the body or legs — not illustrated).

These stimulatory warm-ups help you to remind the brain about the parts of your body that are vulnerable to injury; you are stimulating the nerves in the skin that print images in the brain section that memorizes body sections, so that you do not have to constantly think of those body parts. In a reflex way, the stimulation of the special nerve endings (proprioceptors) helps your body to recognize, in a reflex way, when some parts of you are vulnerable to an injury. After being trained to recognize a danger, a good example of the proprioceptors working is with the back. Many low back strains occur suddenly; without warning, and after only a slight activity, the back can go into severe spasm, leaving the sufferer in severe pain and disabled. With pummeling and the other exercises listed, the proprioceptors are primed and ready to alert the person that perhaps their back joints are in a bad position, thereby warning the person to quickly change their stance or activity. The description that previous low back pain sufferers give is that, instead of their back suddenly going into spasm, they feel an initial warning twinge of discomfort. If they change positions quickly, the usual back spasm attacks are avoided.

The Tin Cans   The starting position is standing, the left foot ahead of the right one, and feet slightly apart. The weight should be mostly on the left foot. Note that the back or right foot is at right angles to the left one.

The arms are relaxed, slightly bent at the elbow. The left arm is held in front of the body, and the right slightly behind the body (see photograph 16-g).

1) Place your right foot forward, ahead of the left one. As you transfer your weight to the right foot, spin on the ball of that foot, turning your whole body, so that your body is facing in the opposite direction. As you turn your body in this way, your left foot should be slightly lifted from the ground, and swept around behind the right foot (see photographs 16-h to 16-k).

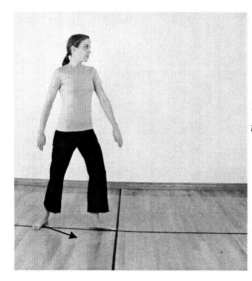

16-g Start position for the tin cans

16-h Tin cans — transferring body weight to the right foot

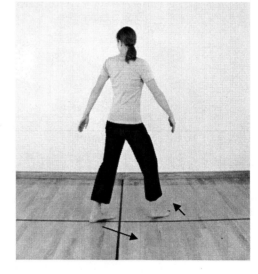

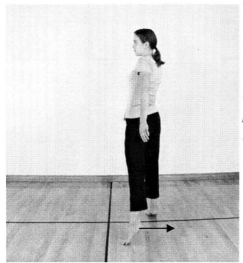

16-i Tin cans — spin on the right foot as you rotate back, passing the left foot around behind you

16-j Tin cans — a continuation of 16-i

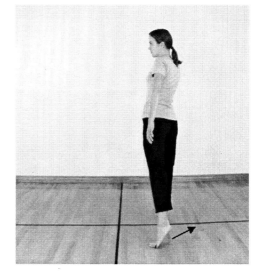

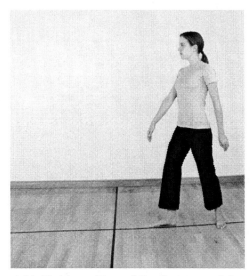

16-k Finish position of the first turn of the tin cans

At this point, you should be in a similar position to the start, the difference being that the feet and the body will be in the opposite position.

2) Now proceed to repeat the rotation, but this time it is the left foot that is thrown forward. As you transfer your weight onto the left foot, pivot on the ball of this foot, rotating the whole body through a half circle. As you pass the right foot back behind the left one and place it on the ground, you should be in exactly the same position as when you started (see photographs 16-l and 16-m; 6-g is both the final and beginning position).

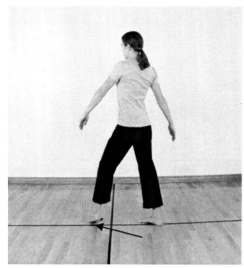

16-l Start of the second turn of the tin cans — throwing the left foot forward

16-m Tin cans — second turn. When you spin on the left foot, the right foot is ready to pass back behind. You then end up back in position 16-g — the beginning position.

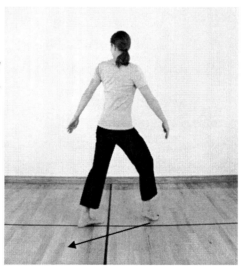

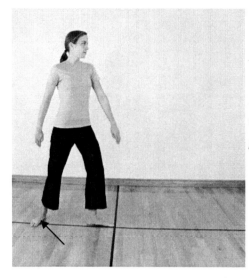

16-n Ending position for tin can, and making room for straight leg raises

All you have to do now is repeat this ten times. As you get used to this particular exercise, and as your speed improves, you will find that it is not only excellent for a *warm-up* but also great for *balance*, as well as providing an *aerobic* workout.

Here are some further pointers on the Tin Cans spins. Throughout these circular movements, your spine should be upright, your knees bent, and your arms floppy, so that they swing freely with your body movements. Your body should not bounce up and down.

To help to be in the correct position, be aware of which wall you are looking at — if indoors — when you start. At the end of one rotation, you should be facing the opposite wall. After the second rotation, you should be back facing that same first wall.

Straight Leg Raises (Kicks) The basic position is standing with the feet shoulder width apart, left foot placed forward, with 70% of your weight placed on this foot. Proceed to thrust both arms down in a forward direction, spread slightly away from the body sides (to make room for the kicking actions, see photograph 16-n).

1) Now, keeping your right leg straight, swing it forward and up as high as you can, being careful not to over-stretch your leg tendons or to lose your balance (see photograph 16-o).

16-o Start position for the straight leg raises

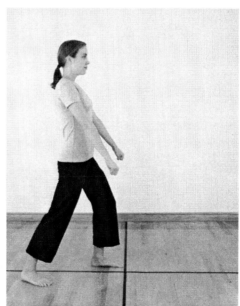

2) Allow this same leg to pass back to the original position.

3) Repeat this kick five times, then change legs, and this time swing up with the left leg.

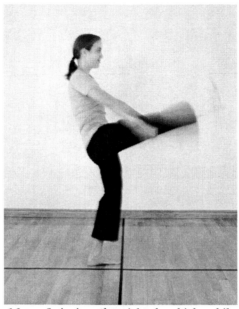

16-p   *Swinging the right leg high while maintaining your balance*

It is useful for balance to keep your arms in the same position (flared out) and your back and head fully upright.

There are many types of activities that will give you enough movement to serve as a warm-up: running on the spot or on a treadmill, or an outdoor run will do. You can, of course, create your own warm-ups from any exercise system that you are used to.

The next part of the *5x5 Mix* consists of muscle toning or strengthening, and this will also generate heat and prepare you for the rest of the activity program.

Chapter 17

The *5x5 Mix* — Section Two —The Myotoners

The Myotoners — For the Unseen and the Visible Muscles

Training of this type, with these mostly everyday myotoner exercises, can strengthen muscle, tendon and bone.

Before external, or *visible,* muscle training is described, we should consider the extremely important issue of training *unseen* muscles.

Deep inside the pelvis are a variety of muscles with important tasks, including keeping a grip on essential organs such as the bladder, vagina and rectum. Pelvic floor muscles have to be kept strong, because it is these, and the tendons, that support and give lift to the pelvic organs, so that these parts of your body can work normally. Failure of these muscles can cause leaky bladders, and possibly a drooping down of the vagina and the rectum, in other words — prolapses. A variety of ways have been described to strengthen the hidden muscles of the inner pelvis, including the well-known hourly squeezing exercises, where you tighten the muscles as if you were trying to stop a full bladder from emptying (Kegel exercises). Apart from the home exercise methods described, it remains important to obtain a firm diagnosis on any bladder or rectogenital problems you might have by seeing your medical doctor before starting the self-help techniques. There are, of course, prescribed treatments available, such as specialized physiotherapy, medication and surgery, for what are called overactive bladders, or vaginal or rectal prolapses.

Vaginal weight training is one of the best self-help methods to regain strength in a woman's pelvis. For the not-so-shy person, a rubber dildo (a phallic-shaped item made of nylon/rubber materials) can be bought and used as a weight in this set of exercises, using the vaginal canal as the portal and gripping part of the body. If you decide to use homemade weights, they can be made with fairly simple materials. At this point though, if the prescribed weights (often chrome-plated steel) are used, it is best to consult a specialized bladder clinic for the brand names that they recommend, as well as advice on how to safely prepare the homemade type. Whatever method is chosen, remember to take all the precautions necessary to ensure that infection is not introduced into the vagina. A non-allergenic antiseptic solution should be used to clean any object that is placed into the vagina. Your local health authority can advise you on how to obtain the latest guidelines on safe disinfection of materials used in this context.

As advised above though, you should consult your doctor for more details on these pelvic exercises. Please note that the muscles that are strengthened are shown after each exercise.

The external, or *visible*, muscle training program is divided into two parts:

The Myotoners — Part One uses handgrip weights. The size of the weights should match your abilities, and examples are any weight from one pound (about half a kilogram) up to fifteen pounds (about seven kilograms).

The Myotoners — Part Two is a system that uses no special equipment (except for an optional soft mat and a chin-up bar, or, if you are outside, soft grass or a suitable tree branch will suffice).

The Myotoners — Part One — Using Handgrip Weights

With one weight in each hand, take up the correct stance for this exercise by standing upright, with the feet shoulder width apart.

Flying With your arms hanging by your sides, simply raise your arms out and up as high as you can, allow them to drop slowly to your sides, then slowly raise them up again as if you were flapping a pair of wings (see photograph 17-a).

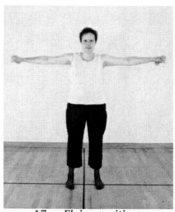

17-a Flying position

Repeat this ten times (the deltoid and supraspinatus muscles are strengthened here).

Bell-ringing Raise both arms straight out in front of you, so that your weighted hands are almost touching. Now, with slow alternating movements, raise the weights up and down, as if you are pulling ropes hanging from a bell tower, or, if you like to think of yourself as being on the farm, milking a cow (see photographs 17-b and 17-c). As you practise bell-ringing or cow-milking, the pectoral, deltoid and other shoulder muscles are being strengthened.

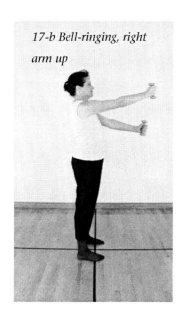

17-b Bell-ringing, right arm up

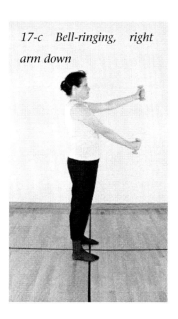

17-c Bell-ringing, right arm down

Windmills These actions are where you have one arm rotating clockwise, alternating with the other arm rotating anticlockwise. For the *right arm*, with the right hand at the level of the left side of your waist, elbow slightly bent, slowly raise the arm upward (see photographs 17-d and 17-e). As the arm rises, slowly bring it across in front of you, brushing close to your face. Slowly, in a circular fashion, drop the hand down to the right side of your body (see photograph 17-f), only to draw it across to waist level to start the circular movement again. With these right arm movements, the hand weight will travel in a clockwise direction. After the clockwise movement with the right arm, perform the same action with the *left arm*. You will see that the arm will move in an anti-clockwise direction (see photographs 17-g to 17-i). By alternating these actions five times for each side, you will, of course, do ten windmills. If performed correctly, this activity should strengthen the pectoral muscles, especially if you allow the weight to drop slowly as it descends to the opposite side of the body. You should be able to feel the hardening of the pectoral, or wing, muscles.

You will note that there is nothing unusual about these strengthening exercises; they are simply a series of movements in various directions that are intended to strengthen different groups of muscles.

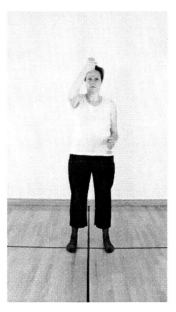

17-d   Windmills
starting position

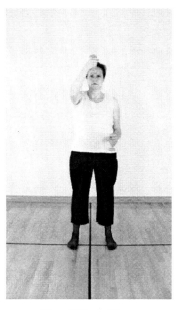

17-e   Windmills   —
raising of the right
hand upward

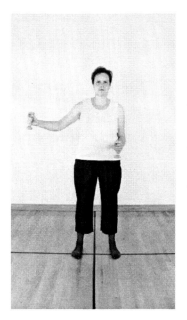

17-f The right hand has been
raised up above the head and
then   turned   in   a   circular
manner out and then down to
the outside of the body in this
windmills action

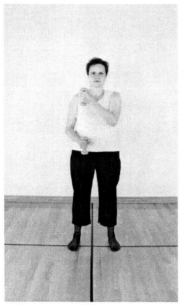

17-g Windmills — start with the left hand, but the rotation is in the opposite direction

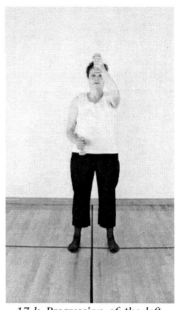

17-h Progression of the left hand windmill rotation

17-i Left-handed windmill position with the weight at the level of the waist

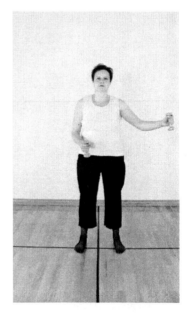

A lot more myotoners could be described here, but it is more important to emphasize the skills of fall injury prevention, see Section Five of the *5x5 Mix*.

Many books or gym facilities have a variety of systems that show one how to strengthen each muscle group. Other muscles that need training are the thighs, the calf muscles, the biceps/triceps, the forearms, the neck/spine, the hands and feet, and, of course, the abdomen and back. Some of these are described below, and some are not.

The main point of this chapter is to emphasize the need to tone muscles to help in the injury prevention plan (this includes the padding effect of muscle). For variety in muscle toning, special elastic bands or similar resistance equipment can be used in this use-of-weights chapter — an idea that is certainly not new. In the late 1800s, long elastic ropes were recommended for muscle toning, and this form of exercise was demonstrated by women for women, and it went by the name of the Whiting exercise system.

You will see from the next few parts of the *5x5 Mix* that special equipment is not necessary to tone muscles and to strengthen tendons.

The Myotoners — Part Two — No Weights

These activities will strengthen the wrists, arms, abdominal muscles, hips and thighs.

Push-up Varieties There are two types of push-ups: the full type, where the whole body weight is taken by the arms and feet; and the half load, with the legs bent at the knees, where the knees and the arms take the body weight (see photograph 17-j, showing the full push-up).

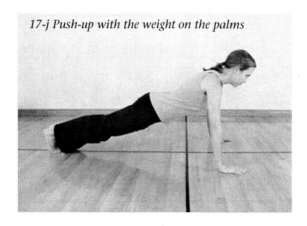

17-j Push-up with the weight on the palms

Note: Full push-ups were demonstrated by women for women to practice as an exercise in the late 1800s.

The ability to support at least your upper body weight on your outstretched arm is a basic need in your body protection, and critical to landing in a safe way from many falling situations.

If you cannot, for any reason, get down on the floor, then an alternative way to carry out a push-up would be to stand facing a countertop, heavy table or similar structure that is sturdy enough to hold your leaning weight.

Try the following. Stand about one yard (about one meter) from the surface of the chosen structure, place your palms on the surface, and then lean forward to allow your arms to hold the weight of your upper body. Lean as far forward as possible by flexing the elbows, and then push yourself back to an upright position by straightening your arms. Repeat this action five or ten times every other day. Then, when your arms feel stronger, you can progress by standing farther away from the furniture or counter surface.

These are called standing push-aways because they can even be practised standing against a wall.

There are many varieties of push-up technique; three are as follows:

On the backs of the wrists, which is to be avoided, of course, if you suffer wrist arthritis (see photograph 17-k).

On the knuckles of the fist, which is a variety of push-up that is uncomfortable at first but gets easier with practice (see photograph 17-l).

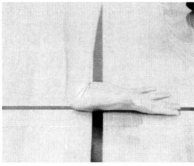
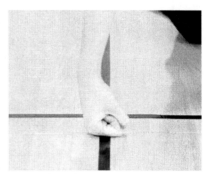

17-k Position for the push-up with the weight on the back of the wrist

17-l Push-up on the knuckles

A third push-up type can be tried as soon as the wrists have been strengthened with the basic methods. In the full push-up position on the palms of the hand, simply straighten one leg and raise it up off the ground. The action of raising one leg off the ground will put more force into the wrists, thus stimulating further tendon strengthening. It is not a bad balance exercise either.

An alternative to this one-leg-raise-type push-up is the one-arm push-up. The one-arm push-up is not easy, but a mild form of it can be. From the basic full push-up position, lift one arm up, so that you are balancing on the other wrist/arm. Instead of pushing up and down, just switch your weight from one arm to the other. Developing the ability to support your upper body weight on one wrist is an even better way than a regular push-up to prevent wrist trauma in a fall to the ground.

Regular Crunches These can be done when lying on your back, knees bent, a pillow under your neck, and gripping both hands behind your head/neck (see photographs 17-m and 17-n).

17-m Crunches — start position

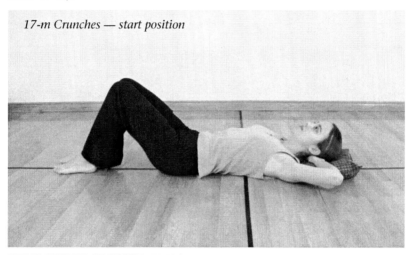

17-n Raising the body in the crunches

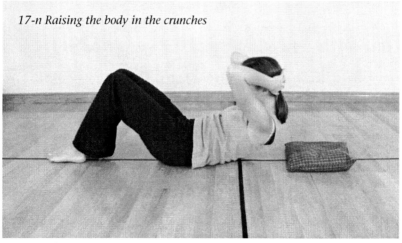

When raising upward into a sit-up position, moving only three inches or so (about eight centimeters) can achieve the necessary muscle action.

Regular crunches variety one: As you raise up, aim your right elbow to your left knee; then raise your upper body up and straight ahead to both knees; and then follow this by raising your body up, aiming your left elbow to your right knee.

Repeat these three actions at least five times to achieve a balanced toning of the whole abdomen, including the lower muscles of the *front* of the spine.

Regular crunches variety two: A more challenging sit-up is where, from the lying on the back position, both straightened legs are raised. The legs are opened, then, holding them in the raised position, sit up with both arms straight and palms together. As you sit up, aim your hands straight ahead between your raised open legs.

Repeat these advanced sit-up actions as many times as you can. I suggest ten to fifteen times.

This type of sit-up is actually a combination of a regular abdominal crunch and a reverse abdominal crunch. The reverse crunch is described next.

Reverse Crunches In this great abdominal toner, you can start in the same way as the regular type of sit-up. Basically, you lie on your back, and then work/move your raised legs in different ways.

Reverse crunches variety one: With your legs outstretched, raise them up and down, alternating left with right. Repeat ten times (see photographs 17-o and 17-p).

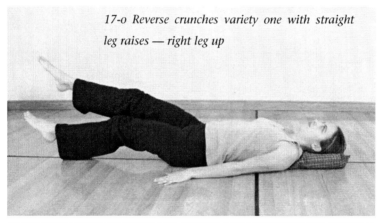

17-o Reverse crunches variety one with straight leg raises — right leg up

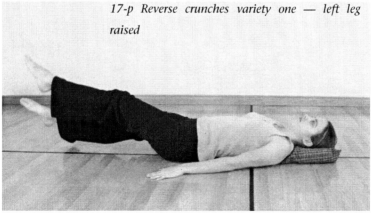

17-p Reverse crunches variety one — left leg raised

Reverse crunches variety two: With your legs outstretched, bend your knees, and then draw both knees toward the chest. Straighten the legs again, and then repeat the process ten times (see photographs 17-q and 17-r).

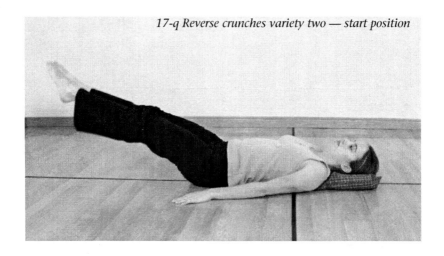

17-q Reverse crunches variety two — start position

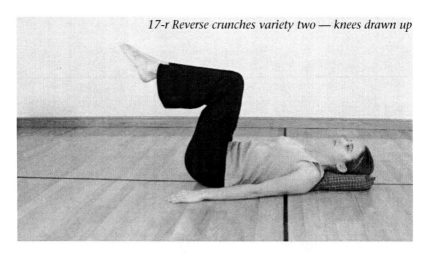

17-r Reverse crunches variety two — knees drawn up

There are many varieties of the reverse abdominal crunch, as there are with all the exercises outlined in this book. But for those people who have trouble getting up from and down to the floor surface, the reverse crunch can be carried out sitting in a chair. As you sit in a chair, extend both your legs out straight and raise your feet off the floor just a few inches or centimeters, and then drop them to the floor again. Repeat this movement as often as you can.

When raising your legs up and down, you will notice that the abdominal muscles are being used; moreover, you will become aware that they are tightening with each leg lifting action.

Hip Region These simple four-direction leg movements are known to help strengthen the hip region muscles, and are also thought to help the hip to resist fractures in a fall (see knee walking action in Section Four of the *5x5 Mix* for an unusual hip toner). Stand on one leg, allowing the other to hang free. Check that your balance is secure.

Step one: Raise the straightened free leg out in front of you. Take it as high as you can, allow it to slowly drop back down, without touching the ground, and then raise it up again. These actions are called *hip flexions,* and should be repeated ten times (see photograph 17-s).

Step two: Pass that same leg straight back, in the opposite direction, so that it is raised back out behind you. Raise the straight leg up behind you, allow it to drop to just above the ground, and then raise it back up again.

These actions are called *hip extensions.* Repeat at least ten times (see photograph 17-t).

Step three: With your body weight on the same leg, raise that same leg straight out sideways, away from your body as far as you can. Allow it to slowly fall back toward the other leg, but not touching it. Now raise it back out again (see photograph 17-u). These actions are called *lateral hip raises* or *abductions,* and should be repeated at least ten times.

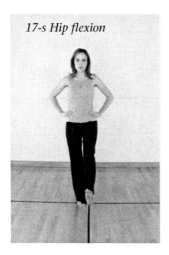

17-s Hip flexion

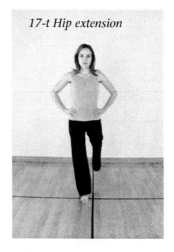

17-t Hip extension

Step four: This is a leg movement in the opposite direction to the lateral hip raise. Simply pass the free leg across in front of your body as far as you can, and then allow it to fall back to the hanging position. These movements are called *hip adductions* (see photograph 17-v).

You will notice that these four movements of the straight leg form a cross-type pattern, as if the legs are being moved north, south, east and west.

Now switch legs and repeat these actions to benefit the other hip. If you wish to add resistance to this activity, you can add elastic bands (available from exercise equipment shops) or you can fit ankle weights.

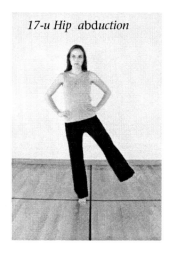

17-u Hip abduction

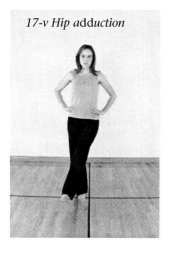

17-v Hip adduction

Partial or Full Chin-ups Chin-up techniques do help to tone those tendons with muscles that are damaged in what are called traction-type injuries. To reduce your risk of traction-type injuries, the addition of chin-ups to any exercise system is well worth the effort. While practising the chin-up methods, you can take the full weight off your feet, or simply pull up with your arms, feet still touching the ground, so that your body weight is shared between your handgrip and your feet (see photographs 17-w and 17-x).

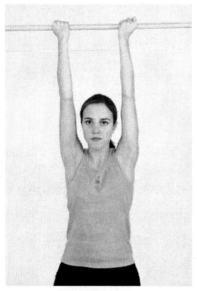

17-w Chin-up

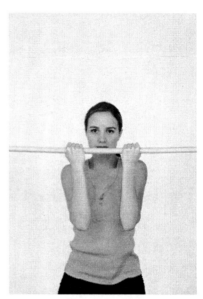

17-x Chin-up

Crawling Activities These essential ground friendly exercises are mentioned here but will be shown in detail in the sections where the floor mats are used, namely the chapters that deal with stability, balance and posture, and body landing skills. Try the Baby crawls and the Spider or Gorilla crawls. They can be quite a challenge!

By the end of this section of exercises, your body should be warmed adequately enough to proceed with the stretches and the *ground reflex skills* training.

Chapter 18

The *5x5 Mix* — Section Three — Stretch and Pull

All types of controlled body stretching are a wonderful way to relax and feel your body parts connecting with each other. You will uncover tight spots in the muscles and often release them. Perform all stretches in a gentle manner, and breathe slowly as you carry out these calming routines.

The Neck — Sitting or Standing Position

Place your hands behind your head, then gently pull forward and down.

Hold in this position for five seconds. Release your head back to the upright position, then repeat five times (see photographs 18-a and 18-b).

Next, place your left hand to the left side of the back of your head, then push the head forward slightly to the right. Hold for five seconds.

Repeat this action in the opposite way, placing your right hand on the back of the right side of your head, pushing forward, slightly to the left (see photographs 18-c to 18-f).

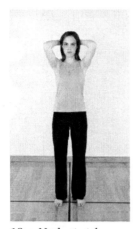

18-a Neck stretch — flexion start position

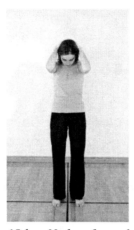

18-b Neck forward flexion

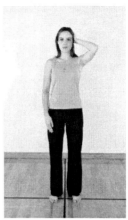

18-c Start position for the oblique neck flexion to the right

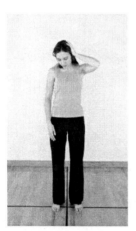

18-d Oblique neck flexion to the right

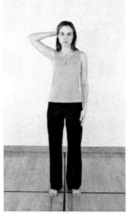

18-e Start position for the oblique neck flexion to the left

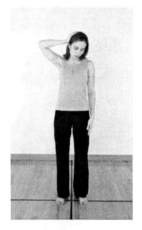

18-f Oblique neck flexion to the left

Chest Wall — Standing Position

If you have trained in swimming, these actions are identical to the arm movements of the backstroke.

Raise your right arm straight up toward the sky. With your body upright, proceed to allow this arm to slowly drop backward and downward behind your body. As your right arm drops completely down, hanging by your side, start to raise your left arm up from the down pointing direction, bringing it up in front of you until it is pointing straight up toward the sky (see photographs 18-g to 18-i).

Now rotate your left arm out and down behind you until it is hanging by your left side (see photographs 18-j to 18-l).

Repeat this cycle up to ten times, alternating right and left.

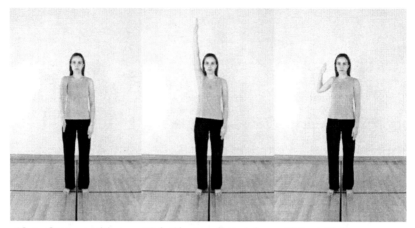

18-g Start position for the chest wall stretch (backward right arm rotation)

18-h Chest wall stretch, right arm raised up and back

18-i Right arm almost fully rotated in the chest wall stretch

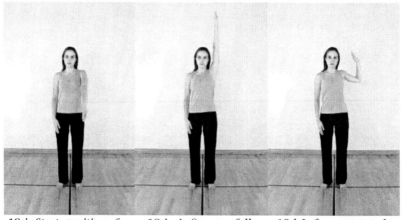

18-j Start position for the chest wall stretch — left arm rotation

18-k Left arm fully raised in the rotation for the chest wall stretch

18-l Left arm rotated backward for the chest wall stretch

The Spine

There are two main spine stretches.

Forward Flexion of the Spine While standing straight up, feet shoulder width apart, and with your arms stretched up toward the sky, bend forward and down to touch the ground. Perform this action slowly. Next, reverse the action, standing to the upright position again (see photographs 18-m and 18-n). Repeat this activity gently and slowly about eight to ten times. (There are many variations of spine flexions, including in the sitting and kneeling positions.)

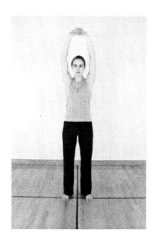

18-m Start position for the forward flexion of the spine stretch

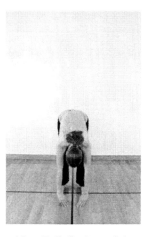

18-n Full flexion of the spine forward — the ground does not have to be touched

Lateral/Side Flexion of the Spine   Keep the same stance for the side bends. Raise your left arm, and then lean as far over as you can to the right, pushing with the weight of your left arm. Your right arm should be bent, that is, flexed, across the front of the abdomen, and this arm will move in the opposite direction to the left arm. Repeat this action five times, from the vertical to the maximum curve to the right (see photograph 18-o).

Now, change arms, dropping your left one back down to your left side, and then raising your right arm, so that it is pointing up toward the sky. You can then repeat these tilts to the left (see photograph 18-p). Try to perform these lateral flexions of the spine slowly, increasing the tilt slightly more with each successive movement.

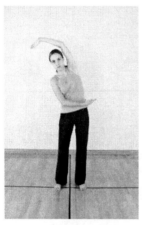

18-o   *Lateral   spinal   flexion to the right*

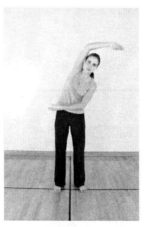

18-p   *Lateral   spinal   flexion to the left*

The Legs

Stand with your feet a little more than shoulder width apart. Bend your left knee, dropping your whole body, and turning it at the same time to face toward the right outstretched leg. Note that your left foot should be flat on the ground, and the weight of your right leg should be resting on the heel of your right foot. You should now be squatting on your left heel (backside touching your heel) with your right leg straight out in front of you (see photograph 18-q).

To reverse this process, straighten your left leg in one continuous movement, so that your body rises up into almost the full standing position, and then transfer your body weight to your right leg. Next, just like the beginning move, bend your right leg, so that your body drops onto your right heel and rotates to face the left outstretched leg (see photograph 18-r).

Repeat this great exercise for balance and for stretching and strengthening a variety of leg muscles eight to ten times, until it is smooth and comfortable. The muscles and tendons that are stretched and strengthened include the tibialis, the quadriceps, the hamstrings and the calves. As balance improves with this body-drop exercise, and if it is performed fairly quickly, it can be a great addition to an aerobic work out.

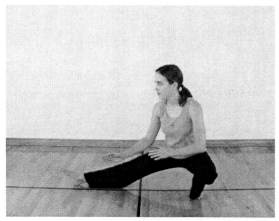

18-q Multiple leg muscle stretch and strengthen exercise — extension of the right and flexion of the left

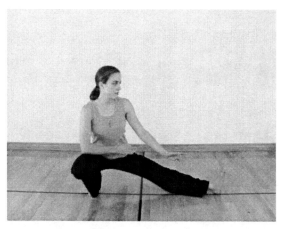

18-r Stretches of the legs — extension of the left and flexion of the right

The Wrists

There are four main wrist stretches.

Flexion or Natural Bends With your right hand palm down, grasp the top/back of your left hand. Push up under the left wrist, using your right thumb, causing the left wrist to bend (flex). You should feel the stretch on the top of the left wrist (see photographs 18-s and 18-t). Repeat the wrist flexions slowly eight to ten times.

Now swap hand positions and repeat the procedure, stretching the right wrist, with the left hand gripping.

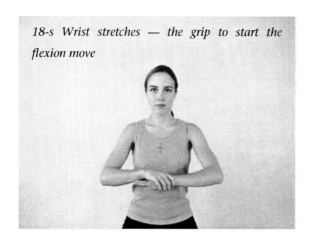

18-s Wrist stretches — the grip to start the flexion move

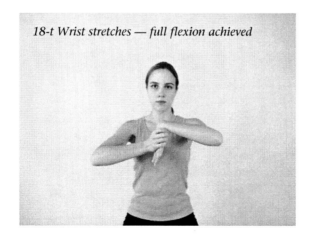

18-t Wrist stretches — full flexion achieved

Extension This can be done for both wrists at the same time. Simply place your palms facing each other in front of you, push together firmly, fingers pointing up, and then push down toward the floor. (Note that your elbows need to be bent.) Repeat the activity, with palms touching and fingers pointing up, first having the hands rise up, and then having them drop back down. You should be able to feel the stretch in the palms of your hands, and all the way into the front of your wrists (see photographs 18-u and 18-v). Repeat these wrist extensions slowly eight to ten times.

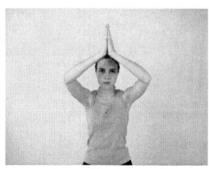

18-u Wrist stretches — start of the extension exercise

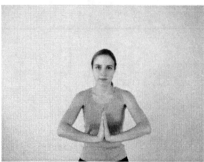

18-v Wrist stretches — full extension achieved

Inward Rotation (Please study the photograph carefully.)

Stretch your left arm out in front of your body. Turn the palm so that it faces outward, with the little finger uppermost. Now stretch out your right arm, with fingers open and palm facing down. Drop your palm down onto the little finger edge of your left hand. You should now let your right thumb drop onto the palm of your left hand, and then grip the left hand with the right as shown (see photograph 18-w). The right thumb will be gripping the left palm, and the front of the right fingers will be gripping the back of the left fingers. With your right hand, pull the left hand toward your body, being careful to guide the left hand toward the midline of your body. If you keep the little finger of your left hand always pointing up, you will notice a definite stretching feeling through the left wrist (see photographs 18-x and, for an alternative view, 18-y).

Repeat the action eight to ten times, pushing the left hand out away from the body, and then pulling it back in again to the midline of the body at about the stomach region level. This wrist stretch is designed to stretch the tendons on the back of the hand and the forearm. To make it more effective, grip the left hand firmly with the right hand, pulling it in a straight line toward your body.

Change hands, so that the right wrist can be stretched. The right arm is extended out, away from the body, with the little finger uppermost and the right palm facing out. Place the palm of the left hand, facing down, onto the right little finger edge of the right hand. Secure a grip, and then repeat the process of stretching the right wrist, as you did with the left wrist.

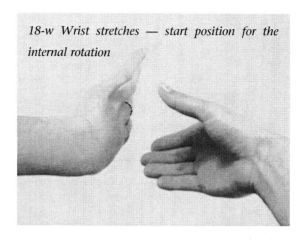

18-w Wrist stretches — start position for the internal rotation

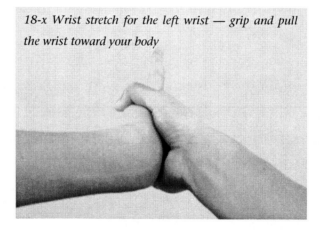

18-x Wrist stretch for the left wrist — grip and pull the wrist toward your body

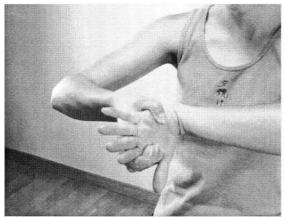

18-y Wrist stretch — internal rotation of the left wrist — an observer's view

Outward Rotation (Please study the photograph of this wrist stretch.) Position your right hand in front of your face. Rotate the palm of this hand so that the little finger side is aimed at your face (see photograph 18-z).

Now, with your left hand in the open position, place the left thumb against the back of the knuckle of the little finger of the right hand. You can now wrap the left fingers around the far edge of the right hand to grip the base of the right thumb, along with the muscle at the base of that thumb. Note that the left hand palm is against the back of the right hand (see photographs 18-za to 18-zc).

Keeping the little finger of the right hand facing your body, grip and at the same time force your right hand down toward the floor, making sure that the right hand descends down vertically, parallel to your body. You should feel the twisting force in both the right hand and wrist if this wrist stretch is performed properly. When you feel that the maximum twist has been achieved in this right wrist rotation, bring your right hand up to face level again. Repeat the same process up to ten times.

Now change hands, so that you can repeat the exercise, with the right hand gripping the left hand in the same fashion. Start, of course, with your left hand level with your face and your left little finger edge facing your face, and then proceed the same way as you did for the right hand.

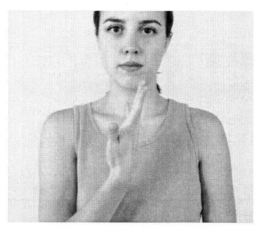

18-z Start position for the outward rotation stretch of the right wrist

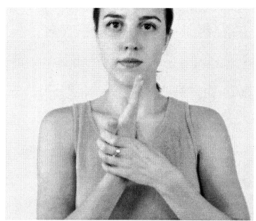

18-za The grip of the right wrist for the outward rotation

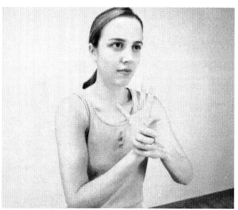

18-zb Alternative view of 18-za for the outward rotation of the right wrist

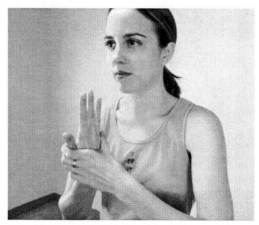

*18-zc As you grip the right wrist, push down,
as shown here for the outward wrist rotation*

The Inner Thighs

For this stretch, you need to be sitting on a comfortable surface. With the knees bent, so that the soles of the feet are touching each other, sit with your back straight up. The accompanying photograph shows how to use a pole to make sure that your back is straight. This sitting posture is a variety of the well-known Lotus position (see photograph 18-zd).

Now, with your hands, grip your feet, and then pull them in as close as you possibly can to your body, at the same time allowing your knees to drop toward the floor. The next step is to bend or flex your whole body forward, keeping your back straight. You should be able to feel a definite pull on the inner thighs (see photographs 18-ze to 18-zg).

As soon as you feel that your inner thighs have reached their maximum stretch, stop the push forward/downward movement, and then allow your body to straighten up again, so that you can lean forward into another action, which can be repeated gently but slowly eight to ten times.

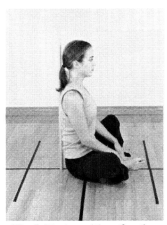

18-zd *Start position for the inner thigh stretch*

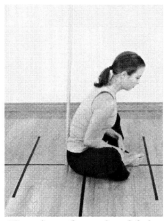

18-ze *Lean forward and feel the inner thigh stretch*

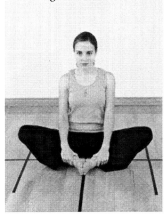

18-zf *Front view of the start of the inner thigh stretch*

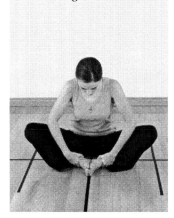

18-zg *Front view of the inner thigh stretch — lean forward as you keep the spine straight*

Of course, there are many other muscle and tendon stretch methods than those shown above that you can perform. The above examples are only a small number to practise. Exercises that stretch the soft tissues of the body are worth doing following warm-ups, because they improve flexibility, which in turn improves your ability to move more freely, lowers your risk of loss of balance, and reduces the risk of a muscle or tendon tear.

Keep in mind, too, that hanging from a chin-up bar is a great stretch routine, as well as an important muscle-strengthening method. It is well worth your while to obtain a chin-up bar to practise on regularly.

Chapter 19

The *5x5 Mix* — Section Four — Stability, Balance and Posture

Two basic ingredients in prevention of a fall of any type are refining posture and improving the sense of balance, both when standing still or moving. When actually falling, having strong balance abilities is a definite benefit, and does help in the whole program of injury prevention, but perfecting balance does not replace well-developed reflex landing skills.

Good balance enables you to control a fall to suit the skills that you can develop in reflex landing techniques. For example, when you fall, if you are falling toward an object, it is possible to steer your body away from that object, so that you land on a more favorable surface.

Practise the following basic — and some not so basic — posture, balance and strengthening training methods about three times a week.

The Japanese Knee Walk or Knee Pivots

This excellent activity can be practised to help strengthen the legs, hips and feet, and to improve balance and posture at the same time. It is advisable to wear firm knee pads for this exercise.

Refer to photographs 19-a to 19-e, to help you to understand this interesting aerobic activity.

To start the knee pivots, squat down so that your knees are resting on the floor surface, and ensure that your posture is upright and that your gaze is looking in the direction that you will travel. Initially, the knees should be separated, at least shoulder width apart. Your arms can be in a relaxed position in front of you, with your hands resting on your thighs.

The idea of this movement is to move forward in a straight line, first pivoting on one knee to gain distance, then pivoting on the other, and so on. In describing the details of this action, each stage will be numbered to match the corresponding photographs.

19-a: First, place your weight on the right knee, with the toes of that right foot curled under so that the ball of the foot is resting on the ground — the heel and sole of the foot will be facing backward.

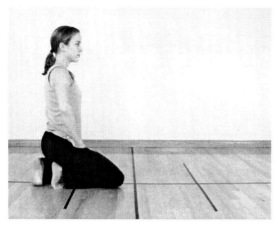

19-a Start position for the knee pivot.

19-b: You should raise the left knee, so that it is pointing straight out to the left side, slightly aimed in a forward direction, with the heel being raised up so that the ball of the left foot is taking the balance of your weight.

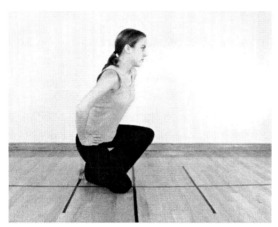

19-b Raising the left knee to prepare for a rotation (knee pivot)

19-c: Now pivot on the right knee, so that your whole body, which should remain upright throughout, rotates. This action brings the left knee forward.

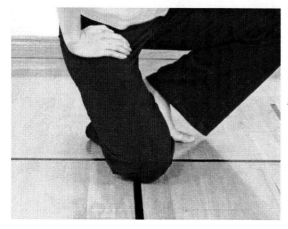

19-c Close-up view of the right knee to emphasize the pivot point

19-d: As the left knee moves forward, drop the left knee to the floor, and then raise your right knee up. Your position has advanced forward one knee step.

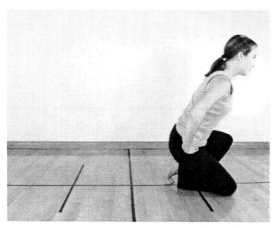

19-d The knee pivot and the dropping of the left knee to the floor

19-e: If you now pivot on the left knee, so that your right knee advances forward, you can place the right knee down, and again the left knee rises up to complete a full cycle.

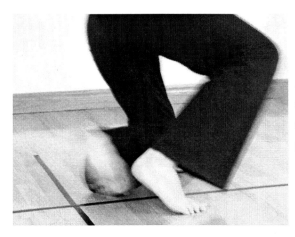

19-e Advancing the right leg forward while pivoting on the left knee

At this time, you have moved forward two knee steps.

After you have practised it a few times, this knee walking action can become extremely smooth and fast. Once you have mastered the forward movements, as you pivot on either knee, instead of keeping the pivot to a small arc you can complete a circle and travel back in the opposite direction.

You can even reverse the actions described above, so that you can travel backward!

Crawls and Other Forgotten Movement Methods

It was probably many years ago that most readers last experienced crawling as a way of moving their bodies. Crawling is a great way to exercise, for balance, for upper limb strength, and for a great workout (see photograph 19-f).

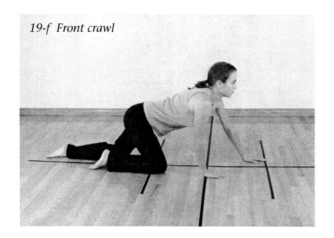

19-f Front crawl

Spider Crawls This activity is illustrated as a drawing of a chimpanzee in Chapter 5, 5-f, and it is where you have all limbs straight, palms and soles of the feet on the ground, and then you walk on all four limbs any distance that can be tolerated by your wrist strength. Spider crawls resemble the way a spider, a chimpanzee or a gorilla walks. This is both an excellent wrist-strengthening exercise and a great aerobic activity.

Back Crawling This is a fine alternative to add to this list of actions. Lie flat on your back looking upward, with your arms bent at your sides and palms down, then lift yourself up with your arms, push up with your feet, and then proceed to move either backward or forward.

The Drag As you lie face down on the floor, drag yourself along the ground, using your hand and forearm power only. In the drag activity, allow your legs to remain limp, so that they are pulled along the floor surface with the rest of your body. People who are paralyzed from the waist down understand this activity well, because this is how they can travel when on the ground surface. Practising this action so that you are proficient at it is worth your while. If you are ever thrown to the ground in an accident, and your legs are injured, dragging yourself quickly to a safe location might save you from more serious or additional injuries. Fitness benefits, shoulder strengthening, and efficiency with other ground activities are some further advantages of practising the Drag activity, along with helping a person to feel more comfortable being grounded!

The Traditional Stork Stance

Simply stand on one leg, folding the other leg up out of the way, and then reach out with both arms straight, closing your eyes as you do so. Count out to yourself to see how high you can count before you lose your balance. Change legs, and then repeat the exercise. Test yourself every four days, and you will find that your balance improves — at least when on one leg (see photographs 19-g and 19-h).

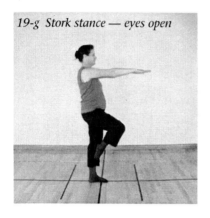

19-g Stork stance — eyes open

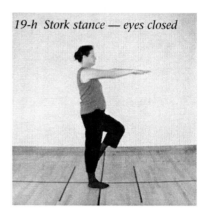

19-h Stork stance — eyes closed

One-legged Pickup

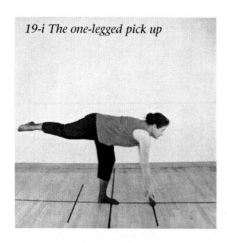

19-i The one-legged pick up

Drop a sponge or similar object on the floor. Standing on one leg (if possible, keeping your head, spine and other leg all in a straight line), rotate forward on the hip that you have your weight on, then attempt to pick up the object on the floor. When you can do this action smoothly, repeat on the other leg. This one-legged pickup is useful, not only as an exercise in balance and posture but also because it is recommended as a way to pick up objects from the floor when a person has an aching back or similar problem, because there is little movement in the spinal joints (see photograph 19-i).

Straight-line Rotations This is a moving balance activity. If you have mastered the Tin Cans exercise, this one is easy to understand, except that you require a little more floor space and it can make you dizzy; however, the dizziness does tend to lessen with practice.

Standing in the upright position, with feet shoulder width apart, place the left leg forward. As if simply walking, step forward, the right foot stepping ahead of the left. As the ball of the right foot contacts the ground, pivot, so that the whole body rotates a whole half circle (backward). If in a four-walled room, you should start off facing one wall, and then end up facing the opposite one.

Although the body turns a half circle, the right foot turns a three-quarter circle; meanwhile, the left foot is placed ahead of the right. Again you will pivot, but on the left foot, so that the body continues to rotate in the same direction another half circle (forward). Now the right foot will be aimed ahead of the left foot, ready to pivot again. When you reach the end of the room, just go back the other way using the same maneuvers.

What you have just done is moved across the room in a straight line, continually rotating in circles (rotating backward, then forward, then backward again).

There are various ways to position your hands for this set of moves. The simplest method is to hold your hands together in a relaxed manner, at about a level just below the mid-waist.

The body rotations described above can be performed as a paired exercise. For those readers who practise dancing, the movements are called pivots. As a pair, the couple hold each other in a so-called dance position and rotate their bodies 180 degrees, attempting to rotate along a straight line. Pivots do need a lot of floor space, because these movements cover a lot of ground quickly (see photographs 19-j to 19-m).

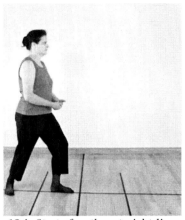

19-j Start for the straight-line rotation

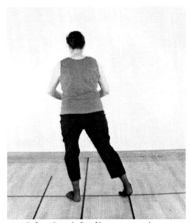

19-k Straight-line rotation — pivoting on the left foot as you advance with the right, rotating half a circle (backward rotation)

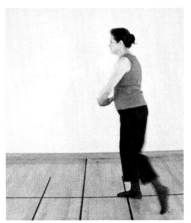

19-l A position in the straight-line rotation where the body weight is transferred to the right foot and the left foot is thrown back, at which point you are facing the opposite direction to the start (19-j)

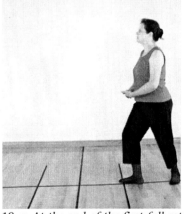

19-m At the end of the first full rotation, make sure that you are in full control of your balance — feet placed flat on the ground and your posture upright! You are now ready to rotate again by throwing your right leg forward as you rotate on the left foot (forward rotation).

Walking the Plank

Walking along a wooden beam, with an upright posture, and then turning by spinning on the balls of the feet to face in the opposite direction is a good balance/posture exercise to practise (see photographs 19-n and 19-o).

The beam used in this balance practice can be a width you are comfortable with, such as a 2" x 6" (4 cm x 25 cm) plank of smooth wood. (The beam shown in the photographs is 2" x 3" or 5 cm x 7.5 cm.) As you improve your balance, try to walk on narrower planks or beams.

Two people can help each other to balance as they move forward and then backward together on a suitable plank. With two on the beam at the same time, other activities can be practised as well, such as leg raises to the side, to the rear, or to the front. As a pair, squats, turns and rotations can be practised on this ground beam as well, and with less fear of falling off. The beam is also good for learning to support a partner while exercising (see photograph 19-p).

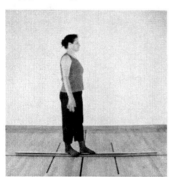

19-n Walking the plank

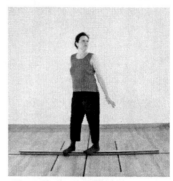

19-o Changing direction on the plank (wooden bar)

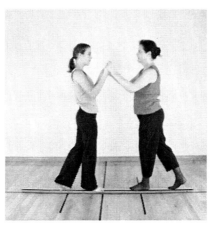

19-p Paired exercise on the plank (wooden bar)

An Old-fashioned Posture Exercise

Place a stiff-covered book on your head, with your body already in as perfect an upright posture as possible. (Check yourself in the mirror, and see the chapter that discusses posture.) Now, just simply walk around your home, balancing the book on your head, and maintaining that perfect stand-tall stance (see photograph 19-q).

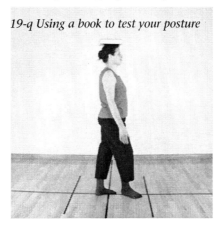

19-q Using a book to test your posture

Just as with the other exercises, there are many more that can be added here on the topic of stationary or moving balance, posture and stability. This is an indoor type of exercise plan; outdoor type practice offers more complex challenges, so exercises for uneven terrain should be gradually added to your overall methods of injury prevention.

There are many balance type exercises other than those shown on the floor beam that are done with two people, and you might see these in various specialized exercise centers. For example, paired balance exercises can involve lifts, and pivoting in a circular motion, and are better shown, for safety reasons, in a real-life situation.

The next chapter of this *5x5 Mix* exercise system continues to help with coordination and balance in a more specialized way, in the form of the indoor level of *ground reflex and landing skills* (GRALS).

Again, refer to the section on posture in Chapter 2 for additional details on this topic.

Chapter 20

The *5x5 Mix* — Section Five — Ground Reflex and Landing Skills for Your Body

Ground reflex and landing skills (GRALS) are a mixture of aerobic exercises and technical movements, and are all designed to reduce the chances of an injury from a fall.

Bobli the ground squirrel, seen in the cartoon on the next page, naturally has an excellent sense of balance, but is here to remind us that almost anyone can learn GRALS.

The importance of this group of basic safety activities is threefold:

First, to spread the impact forces of a fall onto as large and as soft a body surface as possible. This action reduces the shock force to the body from almost any type of fall.

Second, to reduce the friction or striking force in a backward- or forward-moving fall. You learn to transform your body so that it acts like a rolling wheel when it lands on the ground surface. These rolling practices can become a reflex action, protecting both your head and neck from serious injuries in situations such as falling off a horse in a forward direction or over the handlebars of a bicycle.

Third, to promote confidence, and to reduce the fears and worries associated with falling and landing on a damaging surface.

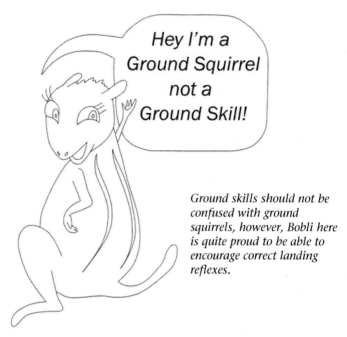

Ground skills should not be confused with ground squirrels, however, Bobli here is quite proud to be able to encourage correct landing reflexes.

Note, however, that full or complete rolling-type exercises are *not* included in this book, because supervision from an on-the-spot expert trainer is necessary.

Training in environments that are more adverse than a gym atmosphere is not included here, but it is mentioned to remind us that a fall can occur in water, on a hill, in the dark, or among irregular objects such as rocks, sharp objects and fire.

Special training is available in falling and landing for people who might be carrying objects such as grocery bags or children and for pregnant women, but again expert supervision is needed.

Two extremely important practice notes to remember are the following:

Repetitive practice of these GRALS is the secret to making these skills truly reflex.

Every time you fall toward the floor surface, *breathe out* as you strike the mat or other practice landing material. Having your lungs empty helps to cut the risk of rib or lung damage in a fall, so it is worth practising this as part of the landing skill too.

To be able to direct a fall is a useful ability to develop. With practice and experience in the reflex methods described in these injury prevention exercises, it is possible to change the direction of a fall to an angle that suits the person's skills. Apart from directing the fall away from a more vulnerable body region to a less essential body region, for example, directing your head away from the ground, so that your arm can strike the surface instead, a person skilled in landing methods often has a better or preferred way to land. A back fall, for example, can be converted almost instantly to a side fall. Clearly, direction of the body to a less serious region on the ground, from a hazardous surface to a less dangerous landing area, is a useful ability to acquire.

Assuming that you have completed the activities outlined in the previous four sections of the *5x5 Mix* routine, you are now ready for the exercise skills, which could save you, if practised regularly, from a fall-related bone injury. Other serious injuries, such as head trauma, can be avoided by developing these same GRALS.

To prepare for this training, you will need a shock-absorbing surface to practise on, a yoga mat or similar surface will work well, and remember — *breathe out as you land!*

Skill A — Identifying Your Arm Shock Absorbers

Lie down on your back, with your knees bent so that your legs are drawn up, your arms are by your sides, and the palms of your hands are facing down.

Tuck your chin in. Now raise both arms up, then let them slap down on the mat. The palms of the hands, along with the soft portions of the forearms, will strike the mat surface first. Repeat this ten times, trying to make sure that the surfaces of the palms and forearms strike the mat at exactly the same time. Incidentally, if this repeated action causes any irritation to the skin of the arms, it is because of either an allergy reaction or an effect of friction. If it is attributed to friction, it will clear up in time; but if it is attributed to an allergy to the mat material, then a mat covering or even a change in mat will be necessary (see photographs 20-a and 20-b).

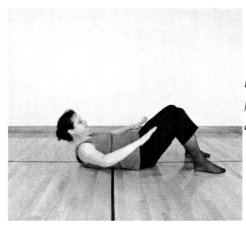

20-a Skill A — keep the arms raised and the chin tucked in for the start of the arm shock absorber exercise

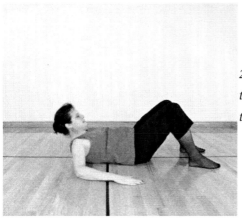

20-b Skill A — slap down on the floor with the palms and the forearms

Skill B — Spinal Rocks

Still on your back, lift your head up off the floor. With your hands, grip around your knees, which will be together, and drawn up toward you. At this point, you should find yourself curled up in a ball, meaning that the spine will be curved, so that you can rock back and forth on the surface of the mat. This action is the exercise that is needed to stimulate the spine, and it prepares your body for the next exercise (see photograph 20-c).

A rolling action is part of a way to spread the forces from the impact of a fall to the ground. Used with the arm shock absorbers, this roll creates a great combination of defenses that you can use to protect your body if you fall.

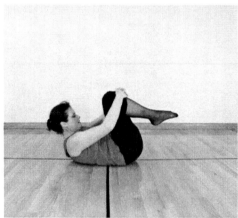

20-c Skill B — simply roll back and forth like a rocking chair for the spinal rocks

Skill C — Spinal Rocks from a Squat (Using the Arm Shock Absorbers)

Squat down on the mat. Curl your arms above your knees, with your head pushed as far forward as possible, chin touching your chest. Now, fall backward, and, keeping your spine in the curved position, allow your arms to stay in front of you. As your spine starts to roll on the mat surface, throw your arms out and down, so that they strike the mat surface with the palms of the hands and the soft areas of the forearms. This slap on the mat with your arms should occur just before the rock on the curve of your spine is complete, in other words, before your head makes contact with the ground. By keeping your chin tucked into your chest, and by striking the mat with your arms, the *forces of impact are greatly reduced to the head and the body when falling on any surface. Practise this activity as often as you can.*

Each time that you do practice this, repeat the roll at least ten times, because it is one of the best aerobic activities that exists. At the end of each roll, return to the squat position in preparation for the next (see photographs 20-d and 20-e).

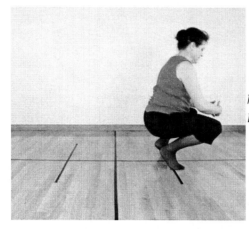

20-d Skill C — start position for the spinal rocks and landing from a squat

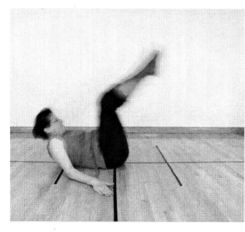

20-e Skill C — the drop and forearm slap in the spinal rocks

Skill D — A Fall Backward, from Standing, into a Roll

You should only practise this more advanced roll when you have absolute confidence in your ability with the squat method as shown in Skill C above.

From the *standing* position, as you begin to fall backward, start to bend your knees into a near squat position. As your lower back approaches the floor, your spine should already be in the curved shape, with the chin tucked well into your chest. Your arms should be slightly bent in front of your body, ready to strike the ground surface as your curved back makes contact with the ground. As you get more used to this action, try slapping the ground as hard as you can. The harder you slap with the palms and forearms, the less the impact to the body. Once this rock is complete, stand up and repeat this skill.

From the photograph, you will see that the arms are flared out from the body at about a 45-degree angle. Note that the contact points of the arm with the ground do not include the elbow tips. Although it is described that the palms and soft pads of the forearms touch the ground at the same time, in practice ensure that the elbows are slightly bent, and that the palms touch fractionally before the forearms. With lots of practice, your elbow tips will not hit the ground surface (see photographs 20-f to 20-j).

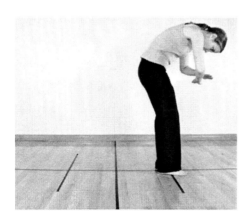

20-f Skill D — a fall back from the standing position

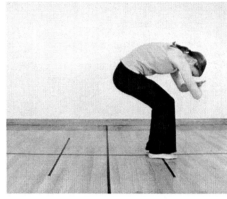

20-g Skill D — starting to curve the spine in the backward fall

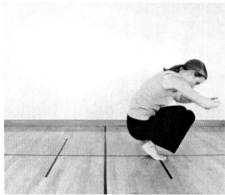

20-h Skill D — the fall back at the squatting stage

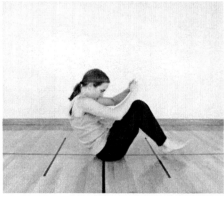

20-i Skill D — backward landing onto the curved spine

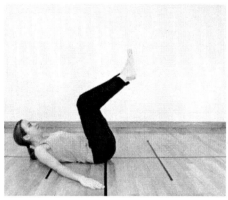

20-j Skill D — final position in the backward fall — the head is forward and the forearms and palms of the hands are striking the ground surface

Once you feel that you can perform these actions without concentrating on the technique, make it a habit to glance behind you just before allowing your body to fall straight backward. As mentioned above, it is possible to slightly change the direction of your fall by a forced rotation of your body.

Skill E — Front Fall Training — Using the Arm Shock Absorbers for the Nose Approach

Lie face down on the mat. With your head back in the upward position, raise your arms in front of you. Now, slap down as hard as you can. Use the palms of the hands and the soft padding of the forearms to strike the mat, just as you did with the backward motion. For each practice session, repeat this activity ten times to toughen the shock absorbers and create reflexes (see photographs 20-k and 20-l).

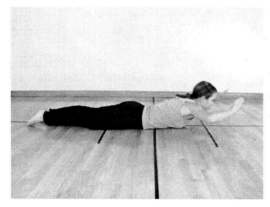

20-k Skill E — low front fall training with the arms and head raised off the ground

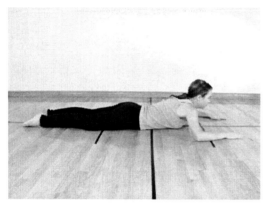

20-l Skill E — low front fall training showing the palm and forearm striking the floor still with the head raised

Skill F — Front Fall Training — Raising the Nose Approach

Start this action in the kneeling position. If you can, sit on your heels, with the tops of your feet flat against the mat surface. Your hands should be resting on your thighs.

The skill in this technique is to fall forward, bringing your arms up to the sides of your head, with the palms facing away from you. Hold your head back, and, just before your body hits the mat, slap down hard with your palms and forearms. This should be repeated ten times for each practice session.

This action can prevent shock to the chest wall, and can also reduce the chances of hitting your face if you should fall forward (see photographs 20-m to 20-o).

As your arms strike the mat surface, *make sure that your head is held tightly back, so that it does not flip forward, thereby ensuring that your face does not strike the ground surface.*

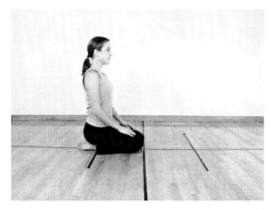

20-m Skill F — for the raised front fall landing exercise, you have to kneel as shown here

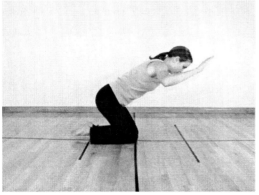

20-n Skill F — fall forward and raise both arms with the palms facing away from you while watching the floor ahead.

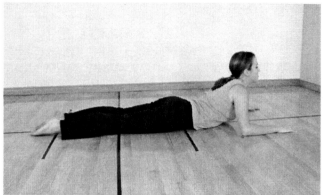

20-o Skill F — slap down onto the floor surface with the palms/forearms, and keep your head up so that you are looking ahead

Skill G — Front Fall — Advanced

The above skill can be performed from a standing position once you have thoroughly mastered the fall from a kneeling position.

It is better that this level of landing be practised with the help of a landing skills expert; but, if this is impossible, keep repeating this skill, each time starting the practice from a higher position from the ground, in other words, from kneeling, to squatting, to half standing, and then from the full standing position.

Skill H — Double Shock Absorbers — Legs and Arms Used in a Side Landing

You will have to lie on the left side of your body for this move. Both knees should be bent, and the left leg should be in full contact with the floor, that is, the side of the thigh and the side of the lower leg, as well as the foot and ankle.

The right leg will have the knee aimed straight upward, with the sole of the foot flat on the ground, and both feet should be touching.

The left arm will be in contact with the floor, palm down, and angled at about 30 to 45 degrees from the body.

The right arm should be bent, hand resting on the stomach area. Ensure that your head is off the floor and that your chin is tucked into your chest (see photograph 20-p).

The trick for this maneuver is to flip over to the opposite side. To achieve this, you have to use your leg and trunk muscles to throw your legs and lower body off the mat and onto your *right* side. Once the lower body is airborne, you have to raise both arms into the air and away from your body.

Keeping the chin tucked in, and as you drop to the right side, slap down with the right arm. The arm will be palm down, about 45 degrees from the body.

The left arm should curve onto the stomach area and stay there.

Now for the legs. The outside of the lower leg should be slapped down onto the mat, and the thigh will follow. The fleshy muscles of the side of the lower leg are the main shock absorbers of the leg.

The foot of the left leg should slap down on the mat surface sole first. The knee will remain bent, pointing straight up. Again, both feet should be as close as possible to each other. Repeat this activity ten times to help perfect this first exercise for side landing (see photographs 20-q to 20-s).

This whole procedure should now be reversed, and then repeated ten times.

This action is not easy to master at first, but with practice it will eventually become quite easy to do. As well, it is an effective physical activity and a great exercise in reflex training. Photograph 20-t shows the final position when landing on the *left* side.

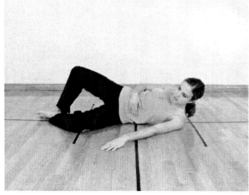

20-p Skill H — start position for the side fall landing, using both arm and leg as shock absorbers

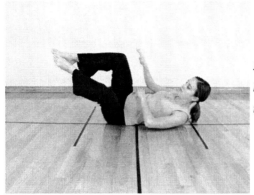

20-q Skill H — throw both legs up as you rock over to the opposite side

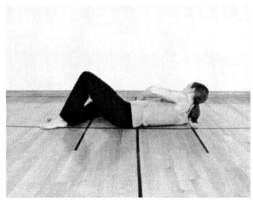

20-r Skill H — side landing onto the right side. With the head off the floor, you have to slap down with the right palm/forearm and strike the ground with the outside portion of the right leg and the sole of the left foot.

20-s Skill H — front view of the low side fall to the right (the opposite side to photograph 20-r)

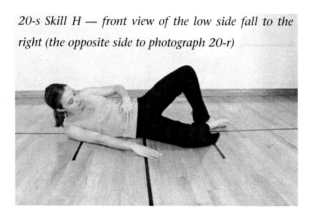

20-t Skill H — final position for landing on your left side, the same one that you start with in photograph 20-p.

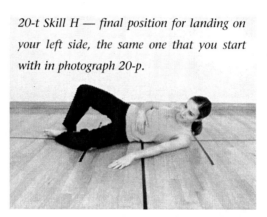

Skill I — Side Drops — One Way To Land from a Higher Side Fall

Adopt the squatting position, and then transfer your body weight to your left foot. Momentarily, hold your right leg out in front of you, and then fall to the right side. The right arm should be bent at the elbow, initially held over the front of the body, and it should strike down to slap the mat surface with the palm of the hand and the soft padding of the forearm. This should occur just before the body reaches the floor mat surface. Unlike the double shock absorber method of side fall, your body will tend to rock toward the head end, away from the hip region, as your body makes contact with the ground.

The back of your head should not hit the ground surface because your chin is tucked in. So, as before, keep the chin tucked in (see photographs 20-u to 20-w).

Next, go back to the squat position, but this time taking the body weight on your right foot. Hold out your left leg, with your left arm bent up over the body, poised, ready to slap the mat as you fall to the left side. Drop to the left, slapping the floor mat with the left palm and forearm as you contact the floor surface. The curved body should rock slightly backward, and I will repeat, yet again, that you should keep your head firmly forward and your chin tucked in.

Repeat these moves, alternating left and right, up to ten times.

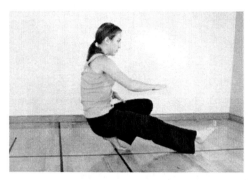

20-u Skill I — side drop starting position (a higher side fall landing exercise)

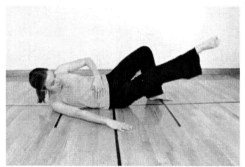

20-v Skill I — as you land in the side drop, strike the ground with the palm/forearm and then the outer side of the leg

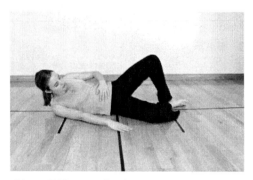

20-w Skill I — final position for the side drop onto the right side

Skill J — Log Rolls

Lie down on the floor mat, on your back with your head raised off the floor surface. Bend both elbows, placing your hands against the front of your chest in an open position, palms separated and pressed against the heart region. Now, all you have to do is roll your whole body across the mat surface as far as you can, depending, of course, on the size of the mat. Form a circle with your arms as you roll, keeping them rigid like a wheel, and you will find that rolling can be done quite smoothly. When you reach the edge of the mat, stop, and then roll back the other way (see photographs 20-x and 20-y).

This exercise will make you dizzy. Obviously, do not overdo this one.

Skill J sounds simple, which it is, but this activity is a great one for helping horizontal balance, and it provides a toughening exercise for this entire injury prevention program. It is also an introduction to more advanced landing skills techniques.

20-x Skill J — start position for the low log roll

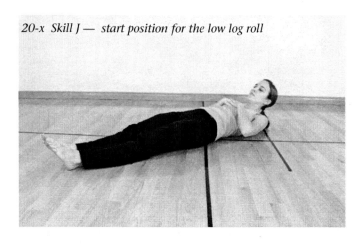

20-y Skill J — Low log roll, over to the left side

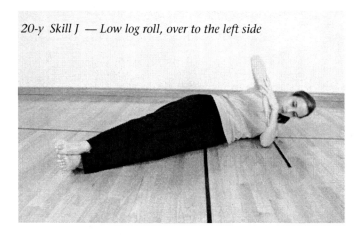

Skill K — High Log Rolls

Start in a position where your right knee is down on the mat, your left leg is bent, and the ball of your left foot is on the mat. Make it a habit to glance ahead of you, so as to know what to expect when rolling forward.

The position of the arms is extremely important. Hold them out in front of you, both elbows bent, so that your hands overlap each other. Your right palm should be on top of the back of your left hand (see photograph 20-z). For all these techniques, be reminded that your body stays as relaxed as possible, but your arms have to be fairly rigid. You will note that your arms appear to form a circle; this is deliberate, because again, as mentioned above, this circular shape will act like a wheel for your body to roll on. Put your chin tightly onto your chest, as always when falling forward.

Now throw yourself forward and to the right. The right curved arm will roll on the ground, followed by your back. Unlike the basic log rolls, from this high log roll fall your knees will remain flexed or in the bent position.

Perform a complete log roll, holding this position, and rolling over as many times as you can (see photographs 20-za and 20-zb).

This skill should now be practised on the left side. Your left knee rests on the mat, your right leg is bent, and the ball of the right foot is ready to push you off into a left roll. Both arms are in the same position, except that your left palm will be over the back of your right hand. With your head bent forward, fall to the left side, rolling on the curve of your left arm, and then onto your back. Again, keep rolling, as far as you can, but not so far that it causes severe dizziness.

20-z Skill K — start position for the higher log roll

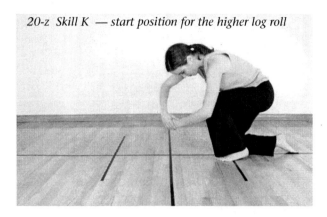

20-za Skill K — as you fall forward, tuck your chin in and allow your right arm to curve as it makes contact with the ground

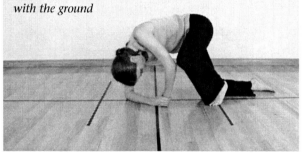

20-zb Skill K — the rollover is almost complete with your arms forming a wheel-like circle. You start rolling onto the right side, but come out on your left.

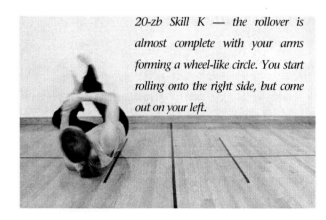

These *log* rolls should *not* be confused with the more advanced *forward* rolls, which are not detailed in these basic landing methods. The log rolls allow the body to roll sideways, but the forward type rolls not described in this book involve rolling forward in a variety of styles.

The purpose of the log rolls is to introduce you to the forward roll, as well as to exercise your inner ear.

Skill L — And More . . .

Once you have mastered them, you can continue to use the above skills in many exciting and more advanced moves. The more advanced the move, the more skilled you will be at resisting fall injuries.

Some horse-riding schools insist on this type of fall training before they will even allow a student to mount a horse. Falling from the height of a horse is different to falling from a person's own height. Some of the more advanced landing skills are designed to reduce the risk of a fracture or dislocation, even when falling sideways from or over the front of a horse.

As indicated before in this chapter, the advanced landing skills can only be taught by a specialist in this form of training, although future books, videotapes and DVDs are planned.

Chapter 21

The Big Ten Platinum Rules of Fall Injury Prevention

As a final comment, please use this chapter as a checklist that you can read regularly to make sure that you will *not* become an injury statistic.

1) Every day, remind yourself that injuries happen to everyone, but that *you* are going to do your utmost to avoid an injury that day. Every time that you get out of bed, say to yourself: "Today, I am not going to have an injury. I am not going to fall over or trip. I am going to be careful, with all my senses *on high alert!"*

2) Remind yourself of the reasons that people do fall over (see Lists 1 to 5 in the Appendix). One day you will not be on these lists; another day you could be — so read it often.

3) Practise the *5x5 Mix* regularly. Here is a guide: Strength (myotoners) and stretching, every fourth day. Ground Reflex and Landing Skills (GRALS), and balance, twice a week. Check your posture, daily. Sharpen your reflexes. Sports such as fencing, badminton or just bouncing and catching a ball are just a few of the activities that can help. Even playing with the household cat teaches you a lot about quick reflexes!

4) Use your surround vision day and night, along with your other senses, to help warn you of the possible dangers around you (Chapter 4, 'Tunnel' Everything, explains this in detail). No matter how many rights you have as a pedestrian, before you cross any road, *stop*, look both ways (as mentioned in Chapter 4), and note any traffic before you proceed.

5) Always be ready for unexpected events, even in your own home. *Familiar places* are where many injuries occur because our guard is down. It is not just falling but all possible injuries that are referred to here, including burns, electrical, chemical, projectile, lightning, firearms, drowning, inhalational (breathing in toxic chemicals), poisoning, and   even being hit by a car on your own property!

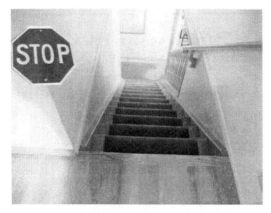

Falling down the stairs is an example of an extremely common in-home injury that really should not happen. As you approach the top of the stairs, and before you begin to descend, *stop,* and then clear your mind of any worries. This is shown in photograph 21, and means just what the traffic sign says: stop, until you have decided that you will descend the stairs with the utmost care and a strong determination to reach the lower level of the home without a trip, slip or fall. Walk slowly and carefully down the stairway, watching for any objects, including pets, that have found their way onto the tread of the steps. If you manage to clear your mind of worries, then you should be able to reach the bottom of the stairs without a fall or injury. Incidentally, remember, of course, that worrying does not resolve problems. If you must do it though, be sure to resume worrying only when it is safe to do so!

Please watch over children on climbing equipment or trampolines, including trees used as part of playground activities.

If you live on a farm or a ranch, you should be aware that injuries here occur commonly and are often more serious.

Intentional injury in your home or on your own property is not just an occurrence seen on television or at the movies anymore either. Being attacked by a thief, by a violent person or persons, or by an animal such as a dog does occur frequently enough that everyone has to plan to be ready if it does happen.

Self-inflicted injuries are also preventable. If you have a persistent depression, get medical or other professional help early, because many people who try to injure them-selves find that they do so with a sudden impulse. If you have a plan to hurt yourself, please discuss it with someone you trust.

In a situation where you are aware of someone else who is depressed and planning to try suicide, even if they say that they have changed their mind, take their thoughts seriously. Many people who are successful with suicide often claim to be perfectly happy just before they carry out the act.

6) Whenever possible, use *safety equipment* and follow all *safety codes* closely. This might be for *sports,* at *work, travelling* (cars, bicycles), or just wearing the correct footwear for a particular occasion. Please apply the same rules to any *children* or *other dependents,* such as *seniors* or *handicapped individuals,* in your life (in cars and vans, sports, playground equipment, and around hazardous situations).

Pregnant women, for obvious reasons, have altered balance points, and they risk not one but two people being hurt in a fall. Practising the ideas of fall injury prevention in pregnancy should be part of all antenatal and prenatal care.

All landing techniques should be practised by anyone riding a horse, as well as wearing full protection head gear (see the photographs of the horse rider in Chapter 2).

Built-in safety, that is, a person's reflexes and skills, is important; so, again, learn to swim, and practise the *5x5 Mix* system.

7) Alcohol and drugs slow your reflexes and dull the senses, and thus should be avoided as much as possible. If you do drink alcohol, and do take drugs that lower blood pressure or sedate, be super-aware of the side effects, and be extra cautious when moving around, climbing, driving, using dangerous equipment, playing sports, or engaged in other risky situations.

8) Get a regular medical examination to check for *hidden diseases*, and seek medical help with any problems that you have now, so that you can achieve an optimum level of health. Understand the ways to avoid stress to your body, and practise various methods to relax your whole self. On a daily basis, try to find a quiet place to

rest your mind and body, even if it is for only ten minutes.

9) Eat wisely. Eat foods that help to strengthen bone, and avoid substances that weaken bone. Diets that help to keep arteries healthy and help to prevent cancers should be on your regular menu. Try to keep your weight balanced to your height, and aim to perfect your physical and mental health.

10) Remember, *intentional* injuries do occur. Being aware of potentially dangerous situations is worth the effort. Certain areas and times attract predatory types. Nighttime, car parks (indoor and outdoor) and pubs/bars/nightclubs are just some areas to be extra alert and aware in. Animal attacks should not be forgotten either. Both domesticated and wild predators can inflict serious injury or death. Falls can and do result from many of these attacks, so being an expert in GRALS (see Chapter 20 and the Glossary) does give you a big advantage in these situations.

A Final Word

All life and good health should be preserved. Although the principles of the above information are meant to prevent fall injuries of all types, it is hoped that, by practising many of these ideas, *all illness* can be *reduced* to a minimum, and that, in general, your *level of resistance* to disease can be *raised* to as high a level as possible. I send out a wish that you all obtain *improved health and have many happy landings if you fall!*

Appendix

List 1 — *Falling Risks Are Increased if You Suffer from These Medical Problems:*

Dizzy spells

Poor vision or poor hearing, or, of course, both

Poor balance

A walking disorder (multiple sclerosis, weak legs for any reason)

Pain for any reason

Tremors

Fatigue

Depression

Anger, anxiety and worry

Attention deficit disorder

Malaise (feeling ill)

The effects of alcohol or certain drugs

A previous broken bone (fracture)

A fear of falling (basophobia, climacophobia and traumatophobia)

Arthritis

Weak bones from bad osteoporosis

A body weight disorder, both underweight and overweight

Diabetes type 1, and perhaps type 2

List 2 — Situations Where a Fall Is More Likely:

On ice or packed snow

In the dark

At home, on the stairs or in the kitchen

Climbing anything (ladders, on a stool or chair, etc)

Fatigue from excess energy expenditure

Rushing and hurrying

Eyes irritated by wind, rain, snow, cold air, dust, or similar
  situations

Wearing loose clothing or shoelaces

Vision is obscured by shadows, objects, sun or bright lights

Sports, especially of the competitive type, and with icy and
  snowy conditions

Wet surfaces, on the edge of swimming pools

If you are unfit

Horse riding, cycling

On a slope of any type

Assaults and being attacked; often you are forced into a fall

Distractions of any type (sight or sound)

List 3 — Everyday Precautions To Avoid Falls — Indoors:

Avoid loose floor rugs, and electrical cables across the floor.

Enable vision to be efficient (stairs, hallways, all rooms should be well lighted).

Use prescribed eyeglasses (avoid walking around with reading glasses on).

Install proper handrails in the bathroom (towel holders and rails are inadequate).

To reach high-up items, use steps or ladders designed for that purpose, avoid stools and chairs. If the floor surface is slippery, rest the ladder on a grip.

Do not rush when doing jobs. Keep your mind on the work that you are doing. If you are worrying, avoid chores that are a high risk for a fall.

Before going down the stairs, stop, concentrate on your steps, use the handrail, and watch for items on the steps that could trip you.

Wear well-fitting shoes, and avoid loose, long clothes, especially on the stairs.

Avoid excess alcohol and medications that can make you dizzy or weak.

Be extra cautious when carrying trays or other objects that obscure vision.

Watch out for pets getting under your feet.

Going from a lighted room to a dark one, remember, your
ability to see will be greatly reduced until your eyes
adapt to the dark.

Be sure that there are no objects between the bed and
bathroom, so that you do not have surprises in the
night when you rush to empty your bladder with the
lights off.

Wet floor surfaces are an extreme risk for a slip-and-slide
fall. Smooth tile, linoleum, or any polished material
should be traveled over with all skills on-the-ready.

List 4 — Everyday Precautions To Avoid Falls —
Outdoors Winter:

Keep snow off the walkways, but avoid ice buildup from packed snow and dripping water. Use sand or salt on ice surfaces and outdoor mats with grips, and frequently chip away the smooth icy surfaces.

Wear warm clothes, use footwear designed for ice and snow, and be extra careful with your first steps outside, because your warm shoes will slip more easily on the ice. The soles of shoes and boots that are colder will grip more easily.

At night, allow your eyes to adapt to the dark, because anytime that it is cold outside your eyes will water excessively until they adapt to the cold.

If you use a walking cane or something similar, be sure to add an ice-gripping device on the contact surface with the ground.

Take extra care getting in and out of vehicles, especially on slopes.

Outdoor steps often get an ice buildup; walk close to and grip side railings well.

List 5 — Everyday Precautions To Avoid Falls —
  Outdoors Summer:

On your garden and other pathways, watch for loose bricks
  or raised blocks of stone, as well as raised, cracked
  concrete, and tree roots, tree branches and other garden
  items, including hoses that you could trip over.

Take care when walking on wet clay or mud, especially on
  a slope.

Wet wooden decking can be extremely slippery, so tread
  slowly.

Take all precautions when climbing ladders and steps.

Look out for holes in the ground.

Depending on your location, as well as your fencing and
  walls, stray pets or wildlife could find their way into
  your garden. Worse than a trip is to slide on a *slippery
  deposit* left by a large dog!

Take the same precautions at night as in the winter when
  out in the dark.

Glossary of Medical and Other Terms

ADRENAL GLAND — A gland that is found sitting on each kidney and produces the hormones adrenaline, cortisone, small amounts of estrogen, testosterone, and some others that help to control fluid balance in the body, including salt and water.

AIKIDO — This system of exercises can be classified as both an art form and a sport. It is a fairly modern martial art derived from the more ancient self-defense techniques of jiu-jitsu (which can be spelled in various ways). This excellent sport consists of three main types, but in its original form did not include any competition. It promotes exercise, self-preservation through this fitness system, along with good posture, self-defense and relaxation. In its practice, because many body throws are carried out, specialized landing techniques are taught to avoid injury.

AMINO ACIDS — Chemical units that join together to form proteins. Amino acids are called essential if the body cannot make them; non-essential amino acids can be made by the body.

ANEMIA — A disorder where the hemoglobin in the blood drops below a certain range of normal. It is the red blood cell that contains the red pigment hemoglobin, and, as the anemia gets worse, the cell (as well as the person) becomes paler than normal. There are many causes for anemia, including iron deficiency, bleeding excessively and genetic types.

AUTOIMMUNE DISEASE — A variety of diseases where the internal defense system of the body (made up of cells and antibodies) tries to destroy its own cells or organs, instead of foreign substances such as bacteria or viruses. Examples of common autoimmune disorders are rheumatoid arthritis, lupus erythematosis, most types of underactive thyroid disease, myasthenia gravis and psoriasis.

BASOPHOBIA — This is an extreme fear of falling over. The phobia is a mixture of the fear of loss of equilibrium and a fear of hitting damaging surfaces and being seriously injured.

BONE — Bone is a stiff, hard, relatively strong substance that develops into various shapes and forms the major part of the skeleton. In life, bone is metabolically a continually active substance, with blood pumping through it, and with bone cells making, as well as breaking down, parts of the architecture. Bone is composed of proteins, minerals such as calcium and phosphorus, and various smaller amounts of elements such as magnesium. The skeletal portions of the skull, limbs and vertebrae are, of course, made of bone.

BREAST CANCER — An extremely serious disease of the mammary gland structure in women. There are different types of cells in the breast that can change into new growths, giving rise to various types of breast cancer. Cancers in this region of the body can grow slowly or quickly, depending on the woman's age and the cell type. Generally, the older the woman is the slower the cancer tends to grow, but the quicker a breast cancer is found the better the chance for a cure.

The author wishes to note here that the statement in the book that fall injuries kill more women than breast cancer does not in any way suggest that breast cancer is a less serious disease than fractures. It is without any doubt as serious a disease, and the worry and suffering that accompany breast cancer are no less than that of injuries. Believe me, the suffering is felt not only by the patient but also by the husband, the family *and the personal physician!*

People often forget that doctors do have feelings, but because of a necessary self-preservation reflex they tend to shy away from showing their true emotions over their patients' illnesses. Physicians do, however, suffer guilt, worry and often severe grief when they see their patients develop serious illnesses.

CAFFEINE — A natural chemical that is part of the family called the xanthines. This potent agent is found in coffee, and is also added to a variety of medicines that can be bought over the counter. Tea and chocolate contain substances of the caffeine family. These caffeine compounds can have a stimulant effect on the body, and can sometimes create unpleasant symptoms such as palpitations and feelings of panic.

CELLS — Cells are minute sacs of living material. They can be seen with a microscope and are different shapes, depending on the type of cell that they are. Each cell is covered in a membrane that encloses many specialized structures, including a solid-looking area called the nucleus. These cells are joined together to make up the various tissues of the body; for example, muscle cells join together to make a muscle, nerve cells join up to make a nerve or the brain.

CHROMOSOME — A thin thread-like structure found in the nuclei of cells from both animals and plants. In humans, there are 46 of these threads, and each chromosome is made of DNA (deoxyribonucleic acid). It is along these threads that genes are found.

CLIMACOPHOBIA — This is an extreme fear of falling down stairs or steps.

CLITORIS — This small but acutely sensitive structure is found in the front part (where the small lips, or *labia mi-*

norae, meet) of the external genitals (the vulva) of the female anatomy. It is made of erectile tissue, and can therefore swell during sexual arousal, and is the most common area to stimulate to reach an orgasm.

COGNITIVE THERAPY — This is a psychological treatment technique where people are helped to change their views or beliefs on situations that cause stress in their lives. The factors that hurt people's emotional health can be from childhood, from current situations, or even from future concerns.

CORTEX — This name is used in many biological systems, for both the plant and animal kingdoms. It refers to the outer layer in any animal structure. Examples are the outer portion of bones or the surface layer of the adrenal glands.

CT SCAN — The full name is a computed/computerized tomogram, shortened from its previous name, CAT scan. It is an imaging technique where x-rays are scanned through body tissues from different angles, as if focusing into the part being examined. The computer of this device can separate out films of the different focused layers of the body region being examined, thereby enabling hard (bony) tissues as well as soft tissues (muscle, nerve, etc) to be assessed.

D VITAMIN — This vitamin is necessary for the absorption of calcium from the intestine into the bloodstream, and from the bloodstream into bone, as well as from bone back into the bloodstream. Natural sources of this vitamin are egg yolk and fish liver oils. The average human adult requires a total of 800 international units of vitamin D daily.

DIVE ROLL — When this skill is perfected by training in a gym, a person skilled at performing it can minimize injury when being thrown forward off a bicycle or a horse. This advanced GRALS exercise is practised repetitively by jumping up and over an object to land in a curved manner. By tucking the chin in against the chest and curving the stiffened leading arm, the body rolls and absorbs the impact of this potentially fatal type of fall.

ECG or EKG (ELECTROCARDIOGRAM) — An ECG, sometimes called an EKG, is a heart test where leads (wires) are attached to the arms and chest so that a recording can be taken of the electrical activity of the heart. The ECG is printed onto a strip of paper and enables an expert to detect many types of heart disease. The section on palpitations in Chapter 14 illustrates an ECG recording.

ENG (ELECTRONYSTAGMOGRAM) — A test of the inner ear that helps to find the cause for vertigo.

EXPERTS IN LANDING METHODS — For those interested in practising the landing methods shown here, including more advanced techniques, please consult an expert in aikido or judo. Before joining a class in any of these arts, however, obtain references first to screen the quality of the instructors.

FATTY ACIDS — Fatty acids are the substances that join together to make fats. These acids are called organic acids because they contain carbon; some are essential in the diet because they cannot be made by the body.

FERMENTATION — A natural process where bacteria digest or break down complicated chemicals such as starches and sugars. Special enzymes that do not use oxygen create more simple substances from these sugars, such as carbon dioxide and either lactate or, in cases where yeast enzymes are present, alcohol.

FIBROMYALGIA (FIBROSITIS) — A medical disorder characterized by painful zones in areas such as the neck, shoulders, chest, back, arms and legs that are tender to pressure. Often the sufferer has difficulty sleeping and is constantly tired. Blood tests tend to be normal, as are other tests in fibromyalgia patients. Treatments vary according to the person needing help; they can help a lot, but there is no cure, although the symptoms do tend to settle with advancing age. The significant complications are depression and a tendency to physical weakness, which are both important in injury risk.

FRACTURE (BONE) — Any break of a bone, whether because of an injury or a disease.

GENE — These are minute clumps of chemicals, found along a chromosome, that guide the formation of proteins that in turn form specific body parts or features. These genes are produced from the parents and carry their features to the children, that is, they carry heredity information. The word "genetics" was coined from the word "gene". For a more scientific explanation of the description of a gene, please refer to a biology or science dictionary.

GLAND — There are different types of glands in the body. Each gland is made up of a collection of specialized cells that make a chemical that is necessary to help the whole body work and function in a healthy way. Some glands have a duct that allows the chemicals to be delivered to a special location. Glands that do not have a duct send their chemicals straight into the bloodstream. This second group are called the endocrine glands, and they are the ones that make hormones (thyroid, ovary, adrenal and testicle are some well-known glands of the ductless type). Some well-known glands with ducts are the sweat glands, the salivary glands, the tear glands and the enzyme-producing glands of the intestine.

GLUTEN — This is a protein found in wheat, rye, oats and barley. In the non-tropical sprue and celiac diseases, there is an intolerance to gluten, somewhat similar to an allergy, where this protein damages the intestinal lining, thereby preventing absorption of fats and other food substances.

GRALS (GROUND REFLEX AND LANDING SKILLS) — This term refers to the whole philosophy of understanding, knowing and practising anything that prevents any type of injury from a fall. In this instance, it refers to the landing skills described in the *5x5 Mix* of exercises, as well as many more techniques that are not shown.

GROUND FRIENDLY — It is important to practise many activities that start in the standing position, but finish at ground level. By regularly practising floor-type exercise, as well as the exercises that are listed in Chapters 16 to 20, a familiarity develops with the floor-level situation. Landing skills involve practising the *5x5 Mix* exercises, and as the skills improve the risk of falling injuries diminishes, making the ground that we walk on not such a bad place to fall onto. "Ground friendly" refers to activities that reduce the risk of fall-type injuries and help you to become more familiar with the floor surface.

HEMOGLOBIN — This substance is the compound that makes red blood cells red. The pigment part of hemoglobin is the *heme* (it contains iron), and the *globin* portion is made of protein. Oxygen is carried around the body by temporarily combining with hemoglobin; carbon dioxide is also picked up from the tissues and carried back to the lungs by binding to hemoglobin.

HORMONE — A chemical substance that is produced by a special gland and released into the blood to send a signal to other parts of the body. There are various types of hormones, and each has its own job to do in the body. Each hormone is produced by its own gland (for example, the adrenal gland makes the hormone cortisone).

IMMUNOTHERAPY — In reference to the section in this book, this is the injection under the skin of dilute amounts of a substance that a person is allergic to. This encourages the immune system to produce a type of antibody to neutralize, or to at least react in a less aggressive way toward, that foreign substance. With time, the person receiving the immunotherapy injections stops reacting allergically to that substance.

INFLUENZA A — A serious illness that starts suddenly and lasts about two to three weeks. Influenza is caused by a virus that attacks the respiratory system; the symptoms are sudden muscle pain, fever, head and eye pain, a cough and severe malaise (feeling extremely ill), especially in the A variety.

JOINT — A part of the body where bones meet and are connected with membranes and ligaments, so that they can be moved in a variety of directions, with the action being caused by muscle contractions. The shoulder, hip, knee, wrist, elbow and vertebrae are examples of joints that can be damaged in an injury. If a joint is forced out of its normal position, a dislocation occurs; if part of the bone is broken at the same time, a fracture dislocation is described.

KYPHOSIS — This refers to the forward curvature of the upper spine. It carries many risks of ill health and makes the sufferer look older.

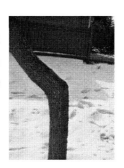

The spine could end up in the same shape as this tree trunk.

LESION — Any irregular appearance in a tissue of the body. It does not necessarily mean cancer, and might be a simple lump, such as a ball of fat that can be surgically removed, or left in the body if it is not causing problems.

METHANE — This simple hydrocarbon vapor of the paraffin family, also known as "marsh gas," is released in the body (colon) when certain types of bacteria break down unabsorbed complex chemicals, such as starch.

MYASTHENIA GRAVIS — A persistent illness of the auto-immune family where the person's own immune system attacks tiny receptors or switches on the sufferer's muscles. Once the muscle receptors are damaged by the person's own immune system, the involved muscle will not function normally. Myasthenia gravis sufferers will notice rapid tiredness when attempting to use their muscles, to the point that they will not work unless rested. If the eyes are affected by this disease, double vision can occur or an eyelid can droop.

MYOSITIS — This refers to muscle inflammation where the symptoms are muscle pain and tenderness. Myositis has various causes, so to find these causes an examination and tests have to be performed by a medical doctor.

NOSE FRACTURE — A painful, often disfiguring, and sometimes dangerous break of the nasal bones. Practise GRALS often to learn how to reduce your risks of this injury.

OSTEOPOROSIS — This word refers to the common bone disease that can occur in male or female children and adults. Described in Chapters 6 and 7, the major characteristic of this disease of the skeleton is that the bone structure becomes less dense as its mass decreases. The architecture of the bone weakens, making it more fragile and increasing the risk of fracture.

PAP TEST — Pap smear or cervical smear are alternate terms used for the Pap test. Named after Dr. George Papanicolaou, this medical examination method is a way to test for cancer, or the risk of it, in the neck of the womb (uterus). To reach the cervix (neck of the womb), a plastic or steel vaginal speculum is inserted into the vagina and opened. The vaginal walls are pushed apart, thereby exposing the cervix, the site of the entrance to the uterus. A special thin brush is used to scrape the surface of the inlet of the cervix, removing clumps of cells so that they can be examined under a microscope. An expert can distinguish normal cells from precancerous or fully cancerous cells. In women who have had a hysterectomy (surgical removal of the uterus, including the cervix), a Pap test should be carried out to screen for the much rarer vaginal cancer. A Pap smear of the cervix should be taken once a year, and that of the vagina every one to three years, or as recommended by your own physician.

PELVIS — This usually refers to the lower cavity of the trunk, but it can refer to the bony pelvis, which is composed of the sacrum/coccyx at the back of the pelvis, forming a ring shape with the two large 'hip' bones (innominate bones) that meet at the front of the body as the pubic joint. In a woman, the pelvic cavity contains the bladder, the uterus (womb) and vagina, the ovaries and the rectum. It also contains the blood vessels, nerves and other essential tissues that support the organs.

QUININE — An ancient fever-lowering medication obtained from the bark of the cinchona tree. It is used today mostly for night leg cramps, as well as in small quantities to create a bitter flavor in some lemon drinks. It continues to be useful with other medications in the treatment of malaria.

REFLEX LANDING SKILLS — This term refers to specific reflexes learned in the GRALS program. With them, a person can react with *learned* movements — quicker than the mind can think — to an unexpected event such as a slip or fall accident, so that an injury is reduced to a minimum. The trained person is able to manipulate the body, including the limbs, in such a way that the contact force is diminished when striking a surface such as the ground. Impact forces are reduced by rolling with the momentum of a fall, by contacting the surface with soft or padded parts of the body that are less prone to fracture, and less essential compared with other body structures; and by ensuring that multiple areas of the body strike a surface at the same moment to spread the impact force. An expert in GRALS can fall and land in a safe way, with some parts of the body relaxed and others tightly held, to avoid whipping effects of, for example, the neck.

SPECULUM — Any medical instrument that is used to help a health practitioner to see a body part through a natural body opening. The speculum that most people think of is the device used to perform a Pap test, where a two-bladed instrument is inserted into the vagina so that the walls of this canal can be moved away from each other to expose the cervix (neck of the womb).

TAI CHI — An activity system that originated in China that consists of a series of movements all designed to promote good posture, correct breathing, good balance, and a safe form of exercise that, if practised regularly, seemingly improves blood circulation, reduces the risks of falling, and induces a relaxed state.

TEETH — These are, of course, extremely hard projections found in the mouth and used for chewing food. In human beings, teeth are important in facial appearance. Tooth injuries are fairly common in forward falls, causing pain, chewing disability and mouth disfigurement. Calcium and vitamin D are both important to the health of the teeth; GRALS are too.

TRAUMATOPHOBIA — This is the fear of getting injured in any way.

UTERUS — A pear-shaped muscular structure, also called the womb, found in the female pelvis. It is the site for the formation and growth of the fetus until it is a full-grown baby and mature enough to be born. Menstrual flow originates from the lining of the uterus.

VAGINA — A muscular canal lined with specialized skin that extends from the vulva to the womb (uterus). It is the lower part of the female reproductive system. Sometimes called the birth canal, the vagina can stretch quite readily during childbirth to allow a fully developed baby to pass from the womb to the outside. To take a Pap test, the neck of the womb (the cervix) has to be exposed by opening the vagina with a vaginal speculum. Of course, the vaginal canal is entered by the penis during sexual intercourse.

VULVA — The vulva is also referred to as the female external genitalia, and it consists of the larger puffy-looking lips, or *labia majorae,* and the thinner more wrinkly-looking hairless lips, or *labia minorae.* The labia minorae pass around the vaginal opening, meeting in the front area of the vulva, to enclose the clitoris. As the labia majorae pass around the outside of the labia minorae, they blend together to form the *mons pubis,* the triangular fatty pad that covers the pubic bone. Its borders are the labiae below, and the groin and abdominal wall above. The mons pubis and labia majorae have a varying amount of pubic hair in adult women.

WRIST JOINT — A series of joints formed by eight small bones located between the ends of the forearm and the hand bones. The wrist joints are frequently injured in falls, so learning how to land correctly, in a back, front or side fall, should avoid fractures in this region of the body.

X-RAY — An imaging technique whereby a type of electromagnetic wave called an x-ray penetrates a region of the body so that an image of the interior structure of those tissues is revealed and recorded onto special film.

YOGA — This word has two main meanings. The one most well-known is the term Hatha Yoga, a series of exercises where breathing, posture and stretching, performed in special ways, are perfected to help promote relaxation and improved health. The other meaning, referred to as Yoga Sutra, refers to the philosophy and the more religious or spiritual disciplines of Hinduism.

ZYGOMATIC BONES — These are bony arches found in each side of the facial skeleton that form the cheek structures. They reach from high in front of the ears across to below the eyes. If fractured in, for example, a fall, they will crush the muscles that move the jaw.

ISBN 141202843-4